DN CIRC

DATE DUE

#45220 Highsmith Inc. 1-800-558-2110

Advance praise for Andrea Peacock's *Libby, Montana*:

"What an extraordinary, meticulous, and heartfelt book. I read it in a single long sitting, which is a tribute to its writerly grace. Andrea Peacock skillfully exposes a true axis of evil and its dire human effects. This is a 'must read' for people of conscience." **—Jim Harrison**

"Add Andrea Peacock's name to the list of great crusading journalists throughout history like Ida Tarbell and Lincoln Steffens. In this age of un-bridled corporate greed, *Libby Montana* is a clarion call to challenge the Powers That Be, and a testament to the strength of ordinary citizens act-ing in the 'common good.'" **—Jim Hightower**

"*Libby, Montana* is a brilliant book by a brilliant reporter—one of the most important books I've read in years. If anyone doubts the interconnected-ness of economic, social, and ecological integrity, read Andrea Peacock's investigative narrative of how W.R. Grace ripped the fabric of Libby, Mon-tana, apart in the name of mining their community of health. And to those who believe this is just an isolated story of corporate irresponsibility in rural America, see how this story is repeating itself in the collapse of the World Trade Center and the asbestos-filled dust that has settled throughout Man-hattan. This is hardrock storytelling capable of saving lives.

"May this book start a fire of outrage in this era of corporate malfeasance." **—Terry Tempest Williams,** author of *Red: Passion and Patience in the Desert*

"Andrea Peacock is an excellent reporter—the reader trusts her quiet voice immediately. She is also a skilled interviewer, intelligent and empa-thetic, with a sure ear for telling gesture, thought, and speech. Best of all, she is a gifted writer and fine story-teller: readers of *Libby, Montana* won't be bored, though they may well be—and they should be—outraged by the tragic stories that she tells about the innocent victims.

"We are all in her debt for this latest warning about corporate morality and the sickening embedded greed that permits these companies to mis-lead their own employees as well as the fellow citizens who made them fat, and even rob them of their lives (as this book shows that W.R. Grace did with its asbestos), should that be necessary to protect gross profits." **—Peter Matthiessen**

Libby, Montana

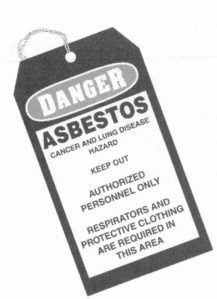

Libby, Montana

*Asbestos and the
Deadly Silence of an
American Corporation*

Andrea Peacock

Johnson Books
BOULDER

Published by Johnson Books, a division of Johnson Publishing Company, 1880 South 57th Court, Boulder, Colorado 80301. Visit our website at www.JohnsonBooks.com. E-mail: books@jpcolorado.com.

9 8 7 6 5 4 3 2 1

Cover design by Debra B. Topping
Cover photo by Lynn Donaldson

Library of Congress Cataloging-in-Publication Data
Peacock, Andrea
    Libby, Montana : asbestos and the deadly silence of an American corporation / Andrea Peacock.
       p. ; cm.
Includes index.
    ISBN 1-55566-319-2
    1. Asbestosis—Montana—Libby. 2. Vermiculite—Health aspects—Montana—Libby. 3. W.R. Grace & Co.
    [DNLM: 1. W.R. Grace & Co. 2. Asbestos—adverse effects—Montana—Personal Narratives. 3. Asbestos—adverse effects—Montana—Popular Works. 4. Aluminum Silicates—adverse effects—Montana—Personal Narratives. 5. Aluminum Silicates—adverse effects—Montana—Popular Works. 6. Asbestosis—etiology—Montana—Personal Narratives. 7. Asbestosis—etiology—Montana—Popular Works. 8. Mining—Montana—Personal Narratives. 9. Mining—Montana—Popular Works. WA 754 P356L 2003] I. Title: Asbestos and the deadly silence of an American corporation. II. Title.
    RC775.A8P43 2003
    616.2'44—dc21   2002156658

Printed in the United States by
Johnson Printing
1880 South 57th Court
Boulder, Colorado 80301

Born by the grace of God,
dying by the gods of Grace.
—Gary Swenson

Contents

One. Dying 1

Two. Almost Paradise 23

Three. The Family Business 50

Four. Mountain of Grace 67

Five. Anatomy of Silence 95

Six. The Watchdogs Take a Nap 124

Seven. Wages of Greed 154

Eight. A Daughter's Revenge 182

Nine. Reckoning 198

Acknowledgments 223

Bibliography 225

Index 237

Hug the Executioner

Small Town Folk
Have Strong Ideals
Love Your Job
It Provides the Meals
Listen to the Boss
He's from the Big City
Hug the Executioner
Ain't It a Pity

Piles of Dust
Lying on the Ground
Piles of Dust
Floating Around
Children in the Dust
Playing Kids Games
Hug the Executioner
Ain't it a Shame

The Jobs are Gone
The Bosses are Gone
The Moneys All Gone
But the Dust Holds On
Holds Onto the Gardens
Holds Onto the Town
Holds Onto the Lungs
People Goin' Down

People Dying, Young and Old
Dust in Their Lungs
Nobody Told
Now People Talk
Between Dry Coughs
Damn the Executioner
Dust is Killing Us Off!

Jenan Swenson-Dedrick, © 2000, Asbestos victim, Libby, Montana

States that processed Libby ore

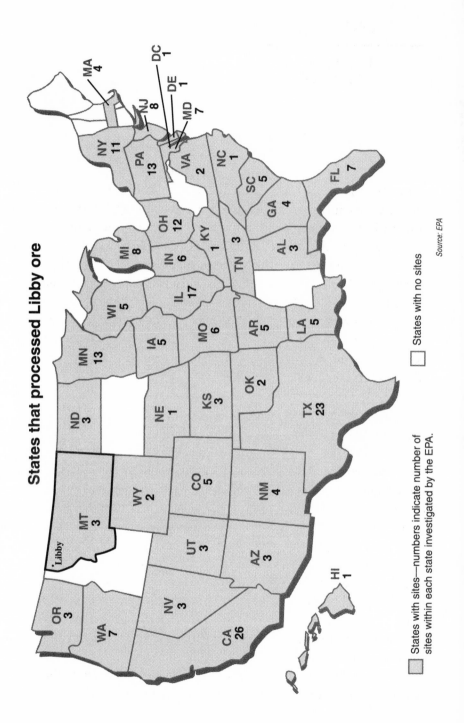

WA 7 · OR 3 · MT 3 · Libby · ND 3 · MN 13 · WI 5 · MI 8 · NY 11 · MA 4
NV 3 · UT 3 · WY 2 · NE 1 · IA 5 · IL 17 · IN 6 · OH 12 · PA 13 · NJ 8 · DC 1 · DE 1 · MD 7
CA 26 · AZ 3 · CO 5 · KS 3 · MO 6 · KY 1 · VA 2 · NC 1
NM 4 · OK 2 · AR 5 · TN 3 · SC 5
TX 23 · LA 5 · AL 3 · GA 4 · FL 7
HI 1

☐ States with sites—numbers indicate number of sites within each state investigated by the EPA.

☐ States with no sites

Source: EPA

ONE

Dying

THE CEMETERY IN Libby, Montana, is not a bad place to spend eternity. One imagines the permanent inhabitants, apparitions sitting with their backs to hills in the south, watching the Kootenai River bend toward them before flowing back north to Canada. The ones without headstones, the Kootenai Indians, named this valley for the river's course, calling it a bow with the nearby Yaak River poised as the arrow. Those with grave markers—white settlers, the fur trappers and prospectors who arrived in small numbers from the early 1800s on, followed by itinerant loggers and latter-day sawyers—would find the town's character not much changed from their days aboveground, espresso shops notwithstanding.

At Perley Vatland's grave, a little girl dances on the headstone, hopping from one foot to the other, giggling, encouraged by the claps and smiles of the adults looking on. Stacey is three years old, Perley's granddaughter, and she tap-dances because she remembers how her granddad used to play guitar for her before he died nine months ago. It is Memorial Day 1975 and Perley's widow and youngest daughter have bought a hanging plant stand for the occasion. They struggle to stick the pointed end of the shaft into the recently frozen ground, then step back to judge their work. Suddenly, one of the grandkids begins howling with laughter. "You skewered Grandpa!" she hollers. It was true—they had stuck the metal rod right on top of the grave. The widow and the daughter look at each other and break down, "laughing like two fools." It was a moment to release the pain of Perley's long, hard death and to look at their uncertain future straight on.

Had they chosen, the family could have glanced north from the graveyard and seen that future in a plume rising from one of the

1

mountains, a great exhalation of asbestos-laden dust from the mill at W.R. Grace's vermiculite mine. The widow Margaret and the daughter Gayla had only begun to suspect it was this dust that took Perley's life. They could not have dreamed then that the mine would claim Margaret's life, leave its mark on Gayla's lungs, and even threaten baby Stacey's unborn daughter. They could not have imagined that by the turn of the century, an investigator combing the historical record would credit Grace's dust with 200 deaths from the community of 12,000, or that a government screening program would reveal that more than 1,000 people here were walking around with the time bomb of asbestos-related disease in their lungs. Nor could Gayla have known the degree to which those events would change her. "I was always a mother first," she says nearly twenty years later. But a deathbed promise to her own mother turned her into a national hero, a woman who took on the megacorporation that betrayed her community and won as much justice as one can expect from this world.

All that would come later, a campaign born of familial caretaking duties when Margaret suffocated from the same disease that had killed her husband. The realization dawned slowly that Margaret's death would not be the last, but instead heralded an era of pain and suffering for the tiny community. But in Gayla Benefield's family, this assault was matched by Margaret's spirit, a legacy of strength and resiliency passed along four generations of mothers and daughters.

MARGARET DIDN'T KNOW HOW close to death Perley was when he got the flu that Tuesday early in the autumn of 1974. Sure, he was tired all the time, and could hardly do anything without losing his air. He must have been on the edge of severe illness for months because when the flu hit him, he went fast. By Friday, Perley was gone, five days before his twenty-year pension from the mine would have vested. Margaret didn't have enough money for his funeral, so her brothers helped out.

It didn't really sink in until a few days after he'd been buried: she was going to be alone for the rest of her life. Late one night she called Gayla and cried, pouring out all her fears. How would she live? She didn't even know how to drive. In a panic she sold all Perley's tools and his car for "dimes on the dollar." She felt she had no choice.

THERE ARE WOMEN WHO ARE born to struggle with life, who embrace the fight and wear the scars as proud evidence of their ability to overcome the obstacles they have chosen for themselves. Margaret and Perley Vatland's older daughter, Eva Thomson, is one of these. "I fought my way through school. Why? Because I had potato-sack clothes—beautifully made, my mom. And I would come to school on a tractor. I had a personality; somebody would say something and I'd deck 'em." She says this with satisfaction. Eva carries herself with a hard-earned dignity. Her parents were wheat farmers from eastern Montana who moved to Libby in 1946 when Eva was six or seven years old. Perley had worked for his father-in-law during World War II, helping him run what was rumored to be the second largest ranch in the state while Margaret's brothers were off fighting in Europe. When the boys came home, they'd lost their taste for farming and so Perley was given a share of the proceeds when the land was sold. The $20,000 was enough to buy 160 acres at the juncture of Libby Creek and the Kootenai River. While her father tried to farm—cattle and wheat—Eva made the clay banks and rolling hills her playground. "I ran all over. Underneath the bridge there was a hobo jungle. My mother didn't realize it but I was going down there every day to visit the hobos. Gayla was born five years younger, so she was a baby and I could get away with all this stuff. It was fun. I really enjoyed it." Their new home was not the picture of comfort: no hot water, no indoor plumbing. Margaret cooked on a propane stove she had brought with her from the plains. "There was a woodstove in the kitchen and a wood furnace in the basement," Eva recalls. "And Mom looked at that and you could just hear her think, 'Oh wow.'"

Now in her early sixties, Eva carries the memory of a gangly twelve-year-old, working until midnight setting pins at the bowling alley, walking home afterwards. Reality is the air, cold and bright with starlight reflected from the snow in December, then warm and pregnant with the lush possibilities of life in May. The breeze stirs a wildness in her heart. By the time she's in high school, Eva frequents the bars in town, following in her musician father's footsteps to visit a side of Libby full of characters, sights and sounds far removed from Sunday Lutheran life, but wedded intimately with the propriety of her mother's and sister's world, so that Libby is a beautiful delicious whole, a community that promises the best of the world if she's willing to take it.

She is still close to her fifteen-year-old self, the girl who left home to marry an abusive air force man, the father of her oldest son. During the next five years they traveled the country, living on military bases in twenty-two states, seeing the length and breadth of America. Eva loved the coasts—San Francisco's Chinatown, Cape Cod. "In fact, the house we had rented was right next to Hyannis, the Kennedy compound. That was before they were even senators; they were just rich people," she says. "The Midwest I wasn't thrilled with; the South I wasn't thrilled with." And, she adds, her marriage was not a good one. "So I came back [to Libby] because I was also in hospitals in all those different states because … he had a temper."

Eva was never close to her sister. Five years was too large a gap in age, and there were all the small circumstances of childhood that keep siblings apart. "The only thing they wanted was for me to be a baby-sitter type of thing," Eva recalls. "She was Mom's last child so she was Mom's baby and I was Dad's son. That gives you an idea of it. They separated us right there without meaning to." From Eva's point of view, the dichotomy was clear: Gayla was the slob; Eva was neat. Gayla was chicken; Eva was the one who frightened her younger sister with tales of the "shit snakes" that lived in the pit under the outhouse. Eva played piano at the bars with her dad while Gayla's bond with her mother would set notions of family at the center of her life. Even so, the sisters might have settled into the comfortable friendship of adulthood had the dust from W.R. Grace's mine not intervened.

NINE A.M. IS A DARK HOUR at the Benefield house. After raising five children, Gayla has decided to enjoy her middle age by
sleeping in, which means company can come by, but they had
better not remark on her pajamas or get between her and the
coffeemaker. Even half asleep, Benefield is a formidable woman.
Quick-tongued and sharp-witted, she can cut you to the quick and
leave you speechless with a turn of phrase, or embrace you with
teasing. It seems she sees through you, grasps your intentions, and
forms her own in an instant. But it's a subdued Gayla Benefield
who lets me into her home this summer morning. I've asked her to
tell me about her parents today. She agrees, but to talk about them
is to be transported. The heat lifts; the noises of the river, of
grasshoppers and grandchildren playing in the pool, all fade into
the background as she begins to relive those years, blinking back
tears. When I replay the tape later, her voice is barely audible.

"My mother was fifty-four when Dad died, and she was left
alone. I mean, at fifty-four if I had been left with no income we'd
manage, but you know, for what?"

Gayla's father, Perley, went to work at the vermiculite mine in
1954. "Dad gave his job to me as my eleventh birthday present. He
had been out of work all summer and things weren't looking good.
He was so proud that he had finally gotten the job that he had
wanted, and coincidentally it occurred on my birthday. I always remember my birthday present that year as Dad's job.

"Mom and Dad explained to me, an eleven-year-old, that the
job meant that in twenty years Dad would receive a pension and
that they could retire and live comfortably in their golden years."

His first job was as a sweeper in the dry mill where the vermiculite ore was processed. Sweeping was an endless task that basically amounted to dusting off the equipment, though Perley had
his sights set on becoming an equipment engineer. He was happy
there, Gayla says, and for good reason. "To work for the mine was
almost like a fraternity. ... Your fellow miners became your
friends. Children played together, families visited." When kids
came up to the mountain, they were taken for rides in the big
Euclid dump trucks. Gayla recalls visiting a family who lived at a

company camp at the base of the mountain as the source of some of her best childhood memories. "We would explore the old skip site, play on the tailings piles, throw rocks and catch frogs in the tailings dam that was directly below the company camp. In the winter, there was ice-skating on the pond and sledding down the main road on the weekends.

"No one in our family or circle of friends had reason to doubt that the mine was anything but Libby's best place to work." The mine, owned by the local Zonolite Company when Perley first went to work there, seemed to take extravagant care of its workers. "I can remember Dad coming home from work in 1959 and announcing to us that the company was even going to offer chest X rays for the employees, for free!" Gayla says. "Dad felt that his health was the company's concern and that the company was going to do everything to keep their miners healthy."

Perley stayed on when W.R. Grace bought out Zonolite in 1963. Within three years, however, he had taken ill. His doctor, Robert MacKenzie, diagnosed him with a heart problem and put him on nitroglycerin. W.R. Grace gave him an easier job: ferrying samples of ore weighing up to twenty-two pounds back and forth from the dry processing mill to the on-site laboratory. By 1970, Perley was so weak that other men stepped in to carry the sample case for him. He finally left the company at age fifty-nine. It wasn't until a workers' compensation evaluation a year later that he was told the truth: there was no heart problem; there never had been. The diagnosis was asbestosis.

Eva lived two blocks from her ailing father, so she and her second husband, Dale Thomson, helped care for him. "Gayla had the five kids; she couldn't do as much as we could do. We were there all the time helping, when Dad was sick especially. I was the one who took him to the hospital for his last trip." After Perley's death, Margaret received $37 a week from workers' compensation, so Eva helped her start a new career. "She figured she could maybe sell Avon. I'd been an Avon lady, so I'm teaching her how to sell Avon and teaching her how to drive. That did put a few gray hairs in, but she did it and she survived.

"We paid for her health insurance. I went to work at the care center so we'd have the extra money because we didn't have any extra either. But my paychecks would go to pay for her insurances, her taxes, and anything else that would come up—repairs on her house—and we would go and repair it. The only thing we didn't do was sewer. We figured David [Gayla's husband] could do something and he did sewer. He did something wrong and it dumped on him once too." Eva did her mother's housework while her sons pitched in by doing all the yard work, shoveling snow in the winter, reluctantly taking a dollar when their grandma forced it on them.

"When my husband Dale was diagnosed, we had to make some decisions. I went to Gayla and said 'Okay, it's your turn. We're going to go and live it up as long as we can and then I'll take care of him.'"

THERE'S A SHIFT THAT takes place when one is newly single, whether through death or divorce. You wake in the morning with thoughts on the hours ahead and how you will fill them. Gradually, Margaret began to live as one person. She saw in the new light of widowhood her place in the world. She started spending more time with Gayla, becoming like a sister to her daughter. If Gayla made a shopping run to Kalispell, Margaret tagged along. Gayla's husband, David, was often traveling, so Margaret became a regular at the supper table. She joked that it was the only place where she could be "served a seven-course meal and lose weight because of having so many kids to serve first." There were still the nights she couldn't sleep and found herself crying at Perley's grave, asking "Why?" with no one but the dead and the cold night air to answer. As the edge wore off the pain, she tried dating again. It was an awkward, funny time. Thank God for Gayla. Her daughter watched out for her, explaining that some men will take advantage of widows, imagining they've been left financially secure. Gayla joked that she felt she was raising another daughter, "only this time a rather mature one who had been caught in a time warp." They learned to talk to each other as adults. What a gift.

EVA'S HUSBAND, Dale Thomson, was management in a union family. Not that he was a white-collar kind of guy. Thomson had been a working man all his life. He'd adopted Eva's son and together they had a second, so he supported the whole clan driving logging trucks, working as an electrical contractor, a ditch digger, an ambulance driver. They met in a bar, but Eva knew it was meant to happen. "Years and years back, way back, I was in Brownie Scouts, and the place where I was in Brownie Scouts there was this piano. And on this piano was this picture of this guy in the air force, you know his air force picture? And that was Dale," she says. "So I picked him up and he was nine years older. We were married three months later and it lasted thirty-three years."

The class differences in Libby are not stark; they are barely evident unless you know what you're looking for. Although Dale's father-in-law, Perley, got him the job at the mine up on the hill, and his brother-in-law, David, was a union representative, Dale crossed a line when he took the supervisor's position in 1974, the year Perley died. "Once he got up there, he got the opportunity to get into the clique," Gayla says. "And that was my first exposure to the little supervisors' group—they'd have their little gatherings and all that. They were really up there socially in this community. I realized how important this little social set was just by watching him.

"But it was tragic because you know the other side of Dale away from the company, [he] was the nicest person you ever wanted to meet." If Gayla was predisposed to think ill of her brother-in-law because of his job, he sealed the deal himself years later when an attorney for W.R. Grace questioned him during a deposition hearing. The lawyer pushed him: After Perley died, didn't he ask his bosses about the asbestos problem at the mine?

"I really didn't know too much about my father-in-law's case until way down the line because I was in management and the rest of the family was very anti-management," he responded. "So everything was concealed from me what was going on." To Gayla, who heard this testimony read into the record after her brother-in-law's death, he had renounced the family and she was stunned to tears.

W.R. Grace paid Dale Thomson for his loyalty by firing him in 1987. He wasn't alone. The company was cutting shifts and staff in preparation for the mine's closure set for 1990. But when he was diagnosed, he got the workers' compensation paperwork to fill out from his boss, Earl Lovick, and insisted that the word "asbestosis" appear on the document. Lovick wouldn't sign it. "He crossed it out, blacked it out, and put 'COPD'—chronic obstructive pulmonary disease," Eva recalls. "Anyway, Dale says 'No, I have asbestosis. I won't sign it.'" A lawyer stepped in, and eventually Lovick signed off on the diagnosis of asbestosis. That same day, Dale was laid off. "It happened to be our anniversary. Dale came home that noon because he had the company truck and says, 'Let's go to lunch.' And I say, 'Okay, why?' What's special, you know? He says, 'I know it's our anniversary, but this might be the last lunch we have. I've just been laid off.' You know, he's been told he's going to die and now he's being laid off. He's fifty-seven years old."

Grace paid Dale about $300,000 in exchange for his health, and realizing they hadn't much time left together, the Thomsons decided to use the money to have a little fun. They bought a new motor home, took a cruise, and were planning a second trip when Dale became very sick. In addition to asbestosis, he was diagnosed with cancer, which spread rapidly from his lungs to his brain. His family watched the tumors forming under his skin.

The diseases caused by asbestos are curious. Those whose lungs form scar tissue, the so-called pleural plaquing, may take years to die. Others react to the fibers with cancer, sometimes a rare asbestos-related lung cancer called mesothelioma, and often die more quickly. Dale had both: the asbestosis was discovered in 1987, the cancer just six weeks before he died in 1992. "It was so terrible," Gayla says. "[H]e would just rear out of his bed, he was like a blind man, like a dead man screaming no no no ..."

The cancer had metastasized, Eva explains, and when it entered his heart muscle, the doctors could not give him enough pain medication. "He did die a horrible death," his widow states simply.

Eva loved Dale dearly, and to this day won't tolerate even a hint of criticism of her late husband. She recoils at the idea that Dale was a company man, reciting again all he had done for Margaret after Perley died. So while the number of family members diagnosed with asbestosis continues to mount, the rift between sisters remains, tension under the surface at family gatherings, a chance for intimacy still unrealized.

Gayla first started noticing her mother's cough in the early 1980s. Margaret tried to hide it, but her younger daughter lived too close for secrets. When Gayla stopped by for coffee on her way to work, Margaret would have her morning coughing fit—a dry hack that worked its way out as she warmed into the day. She excused it to Gayla as a reaction to her dentures or as allergies. When Gayla suggested that it could be related to the disease that had killed Perley, she shrugged it off. But the suspicion lay in the back of her mind as well.

Margaret buried her fears in a flurry of activity. She worked her Avon route until she became one of the area's top distributors. She drove her grandkids to their ball games, took them swimming in Libby Creek where it dumped into the Kootenai River, and often called Gayla's house and invited the "two best kids" that day over for dinner. The children drove away the loneliness for a while. Around that time, her brother Kermit retired and invited Margaret along for road trips with him and his wife. They'd start by heading for Reno and then end up wherever the road took them—a right turn here, a left turn there. And they played games: farting contests in the camper at night, stealing toilet paper from gas station bathrooms. It was like being a kid again.

JENAN SWENSON DID NOT EASE into adulthood. One could say she slipped and fell into a deep pool of responsibility with the birth of her first daughter at age nineteen and has been trying to keep her head above water ever since. Now in her late thirties, she has three girls, all of whom she's raised mostly as a single mom. She is pretty with a broad, open face; a poet who streaks her blonde hair red. She has a deep religious faith she turns to when searching for meaning in the things happening to her family. She works hard and struggles financially in one of the most economically depressed counties in Montana, one of the poorest states in the nation. But she'd tell you it would be a mistake to say she's accomplished the task alone. As Gayla's oldest (the only child of her mother's first brief marriage to a local boy named Gary Swenson), Jenan learned early the value of a large extended family: aunts and cousins make great baby-sitters and playmates. But of all her relatives, she was particularly close to her grandma Margaret. "Everyone always thought I was the third daughter," she says. "There's Eva and Mom, and then I was the first granddaughter. And even one day Mom and I were driving into town and Mom says, 'And when you see your mother, you tell her ...' And I'm like, 'You're my mother.'" Jenan delivers this story deadpan, then follows with an easy laugh that belies the previous five years during which she struggled with the grief over her grandma's death.

"Anytime Mom had a baby I'd go spend the first month with Grandma. I'd spend summers with her. We lived in like four or five different houses within a couple blocks of her growing up. Even when our dogs would run away we'd just go down to Grandma's and they'd be there waiting for us. You just went to Grandma's like almost every day. You couldn't leave without eating, you know. She'd make you fix a sandwich or have a cookie and stuff, and that is something that just continued on into adulthood. I would have lunch hour at work and I'd go to Grandma's and have a sandwich, watch *Days of Our Lives*, and she'd fall asleep and I'd go back to work."

After two failed marriages, attempts to start over in other states, and finally the move back to Libby, maybe the only fairy tale part of Jenan's life was the steadfast presence of Margaret. "It was always a happy place to go to Grandma's, it was always a safe place to go to Grandma's. You always felt like you were something really special when you were with Grandma." She pauses and takes a drag off her cigarette. "We didn't even realize until after she had died how we'd forgotten that. She'd just become bitter, bitter and very controlling. Then, all the disease had left her body and she looked like she did fifteen years before. It was like seeing an old friend."

A fact of asbestos-related diseases is that they can rob people of their lives for years before they actually die. Margaret's cough progressed until she was so run down she couldn't shake a cold. Eva came to visit one Sunday afternoon in the spring of 1985 to find her mother in bed, unable to get up. She called an ambulance and at the hospital Margaret was diagnosed with pneumonia. Gayla asked the admitting doctor if her mother had the same disease that had killed her father, but received no reply. For the next three years Margaret was plagued with health problems: a misdiagnosis of lung cancer, ostensibly related to her smoking. Though the doctor said she wouldn't live to see Christmas, Margaret did not seem to deteriorate the way he had predicted. There was the cervical cancer, found almost accidentally—her first Pap smear in two decades. One Christmas Eve, she suffered a series of small strokes.

As Margaret's health deteriorated, she gradually accepted that she needed to go after W.R. Grace for some money. She was, Gayla says, greatly intimidated by the prospect. "In those days, people did not sue and did not go to court," Gayla says. "You just didn't do that. She was going in for a deposition the day they made her the offer. She was scared to death of a deposition." Margaret settled with the company in 1988 for $100,000, of which she received $67,000—not much by big city standards, but enough to qualify as "Libby Rich." She spent $10,000 on a brand-new Ford Escort, another $1,000 on a couch, and saved the rest. She knew she would need it for medical care. Around this time, she was finally willing to talk with her younger daughter about her declining health. To Gayla this was a relief; her father had slipped away before she was ready. They never took the time to talk about his impending death. She was determined not to let her mother go in the same manner. "I made up my mind then that I would never let my mother leave me so abruptly without saying everything that I wanted to tell her."

After the settlement, Margaret was ready for those talks. "She finally admitted to me how terrified she was of dying in the same manner as Dad," Gayla says. "We sat and talked for hours. We finally decided that she should seek medical help." In 1988, Margaret received official confirmation of what Gayla had suspected all along: it was asbestos, not cigarettes, scarring her mother's lungs. "[The doctor] had never heard of anyone getting exposed without working in a factory or mine. He doubted that she had asbestosis," Gayla says. "After the surgery, [he] came into the waiting room to tell us that there was never any sign of lung cancer." The surgeon removed two sections of Margaret's lung that, he told the family, he felt sure had been damaged by asbestos.

FIRST ARE THE VARIOUS WAYS TO describe what is happening to Margaret's lungs: pleural plaquing, the tissue on the outside becoming a straightjacket with the texture of an orange rind. Asbestosis. But there are more ways of talking about her infirmity, and these are measured by the changes in her life. She sleeps on a sofa she bought with part of the settlement she got from Grace, unable now to climb the stairs to the bedroom of her Minnesota Avenue home. She gave up the garden because the effort to turn the soil was too great. It was never a big production—just a patch large enough for some lettuce and peas for her granddaughter Stacey. Margaret knows her life is being cut short. Her own mother is still alive, going strong in her late nineties, and may outlive Margaret. But sadder yet, Margaret finds that of her ten great-grandchildren, she must choose three she has the energy for and let the rest go. She knows she won't live to see them grow up anyway.

WHEN MARGARET CAME HOME from the hospital after the 1988 surgery, her routine changed noticeably. She had lost all her energy and was frustrated by her body's betrayal. In retrospect, it was the point at which Margaret began to leave her family, as bitterness set in. "I convinced her to start having someone come in to clean her house," Gayla says. "She had to learn to prioritize what energy she had. I convinced her that if she didn't waste so much strength trying to do everything for herself, she would have more energy to do the things she enjoyed."

For a woman who had raised her family cooking on a propane stove, a farmer's wife who had survived winters on the prairies and the floods of spring, taking it easy did not come naturally. One evening Gayla came by to find her sitting out on the back stoop. "Her new little car was pulled up into her yard. A bucket of water and a hose were lying by the car. I asked her what she had tried to do this time. She told me she had decided to wash her car. She was doing fine until she slammed the car door after wiping down the inside. Suddenly, she realized that she had slammed her oxygen hose in the car door and accidentally locked the door at the same time." Margaret had a spare tank of oxygen on the back porch, so she disconnected the hose at her waist and ran for the house where Gayla found her sitting. "The reason she was sitting on the back step was because she admitted that she suddenly was too exhausted to go back into the house and find her car keys, and while I was there, would I please finish washing her car for her?"

In May 1990, Margaret's oxygen tube was replaced with a "trans-tracheal scoop" inserted surgically into her throat to deliver oxygen to her lungs. Her days became regimented. The scoop had to be cleaned twice a day, a process during which she used her old oxygen tube while spraying Broncho-Saline down the scoop. This caused her to cough, a necessary part of the process, as a blockage the size of a pea would form at the end of the scoop and would eventually cut off her airflow if she didn't cough it up. Then she had to remove the tube and insert a sterile one. Plus there was the medication. "Before my mother died, her medication was $600 a month. They have inhalers, they have an elixir we called snake oil to keep the mucus soft, otherwise it gets syrupy. Antibiotics, you've got to take potassium, you've got to take water pills," Gayla says. "You're looking at a full day of doing simply nothing but taking medicine." There were pills at 10 A.M., more at noon, the inhaler at 2. "Her Theo-Dur [broncho-dilator] capsules were an absolute necessity. If she didn't have her pill at the prescribed time, within an hour she would have trouble breathing." Margaret's life diminished steadily. She had always loved to cook, and refused the TV dinners her family offered on the days she had no strength for the kitchen. Instead she made large meals on her good days and froze the leftovers for the future. Once in a while Gayla caught her trying to bake cookies for her grandchildren, but the effort was such that she couldn't finish the job. By 1993 Margaret could no longer live alone in her home of forty-two years.

She and Gayla had their jokes, and at times it was the only thing that lifted her spirits. After a bout with pneumonia that landed her in the hospital, Margaret began praising her daughter as "her angel" whenever she showed up to empty the bedpan or clean the trach. Gayla finally retorted that when her mother reached the afterlife, she was to put in a good word with the "higher being" to make her a "skinny angel with boobs" for all eternity. Margaret let the nurses in on the joke, and occasionally would inform Gayla that "a certain nurse ... would definitely weigh 300 pounds" if she had anything to say about it. After that stay in the hospital, a doctor recommended moving her to a nursing home. She considered this: Gayla was stretched thin financially and emotionally. Eva had only recently watched her husband, Dale, die and wasn't prepared to care for a sick mother. The joked-about "Shady Rest Nursing Home" suddenly became a real possibility. She extracted a promise from Gayla: "Only after I lose my mind and wear a diaper" could her family put her in such a place. It was a late-night promise, but one she knew she could count on her daughter to keep.

The smallest incidents would almost be funny if it weren't for the dire consequences. She called Gayla one day when her oxygen compressor seemed to be on the blink—she had set it as high as she could, but was still experiencing hot flashes from the lack of air. Gayla drove over and began checking the apparatus inch by inch. Finally she found a section of the hose filled with holes—one of her mother's two cats had chewed it to pieces.

IT TOOK SEVENTEEN MONTHS FOR Margaret to die, and her care during that time was a group effort. The family hired nurses to stay during the week—day and night—at the mobile home court where Margaret now lived three minutes from Gayla's house. "Actually, five minutes if I took time to put on shoes and drive safely," Gayla says. "But three minutes was the record from a dead sleep." On the weekends and in between shifts, the family filled in. For the kids it was precious time with their great-grandma. Amy Boeck, Jenan's oldest daughter, recalls spending hours playing cards—Go Fish, mainly—and talking. But for the adults it was grueling.

"The only control she had in her life was over her caregivers," Jenan says. "One day [my sister-in-law] Amber was down there working and I stopped in to visit. Within fifteen minutes she had me and Amber winded. 'You need to do this, you need to do that.' You know, the caregivers would leave every night just in tears because Grandma was so controlling and so bossy."

Gayla kept a phone by her bed and instructed her mother to call even if she was just lonely. "There were nights when she would call just to hear my voice. She didn't want to talk about anything in particular. Generally, I would get some clothes on and go in and sit with her.

"Those were the nights we talked about dying. She was not frightened of death, she was only frightened of the way it would occur. She had watched Dad slowly fight for every breath for three days. She didn't want that. She insisted that she not be resuscitated.

"Mom always said that with her luck, she would be brought back to life after a very comfortable death. She told me that she prayed at night to not wake up." Of all Margaret's requests, this was one of the hardest for Gayla. There were days when Margaret started to slip away, when her oxygen and medications were out of balance. Gayla could have simply let her go to sleep for good; instead she found herself calling the doctor. Why? "Well, you know, to me it was murder to deny help when help was available," she says. It won't happen again. "Knowing now what I knew then, the next person in my family that would happen to, I would simply do that. I would probably let her suffocate."

For months, Margaret had been unable to control her body temperature. She would get the chills when the thermostat read 90 degrees, and other times the hot flashes—a side effect of oxygen deprivation—would hit and she would wrap up in a sheet from the freezer. The 1995 summer forest fire season was agony. Asbestosis afflicts its victims with claustrophobia, and as the disease progresses many people have a hard time sitting in a room with the windows shut. "All I could do was duct-tape wet towels over the open windows," Gayla says. "Within a few hours, the towels were brown with smoke and would have to be changed. We managed, but the exposure to the smoke weakened her lungs even more."

The family tried to keep Margaret involved in life by bringing their world to her. One Christmas they made a video of the festivities. She told them to turn it off because it was too painful to watch. Margaret was leaving them. She became jealous of Gayla's freedom to do the simplest things: to go shopping or take a drive. She reacted to her own growing helplessness by manipulating those around her. Gayla took herself off call for only a few hours each week to go bowling in a league. As Margaret's resentment grew, she started calling for help with her trach just as she knew Gayla was leaving for the bowling alley. During a particularly rough hospital stay, she called the Benefield home twenty-one times in one day. Their special mother-daughter talks ceased. "She didn't want to hear about my life. She didn't feel it necessary to share hers," Gayla recalls. "By the summer of 1995 the mother who had once been my best friend was no longer there."

MARGARET WAS ANGRY—furious with Perley, her beloved husband, for dying and leaving her sick and alone, for those wild years when he seemed happier at the bars, playing music and drinking too much, than at home. She shouted curses at him during the night for bringing home that dust on his clothes. When her anger was cold and lucid she blamed the company, W.R. Grace, and its bosses—damn Earl Lovick to hell—for killing her husband and squeezing her life away with every breath. In private she might have cried for all that was lost. But on top of it all, she had precious little privacy these days—she needed too much help to be left alone for long. She knew she was unpleasant to be around, but it hardly seemed to matter—the world she had lived in was gone. Her children and grandchildren, even her cats, passed through the bedroom like ghosts.

FINANCIALLY THE BENEFIELDS were nearly broken. Margaret's basic care reached $3,000 a month. Gayla cashed in a $10,000 CD her mother had given her and paid it out for four months' worth of nursing care. Eva's CD paid for another four months. The family could save almost $3 per can of Broncho-Saline to clean Margaret's trach by driving 90 miles down a mountain road to Kalispell, so whenever anyone made the trip they were instructed to buy out the store. Gayla finally mortgaged Margaret's mobile home for $15,000, and Eva chipped in another $10,000. Thanks to a delicate balancing act of thrift and resourcefulness, the last seventeen months of Margaret's life cost only $50,000. In anger and desperation Gayla started shopping around for lawyers. When she found one who said he'd bring a wrongful death suit, she brought the news home to her mother. "She thought it was wonderful. She said, 'I hope we get those bastards,'" Gayla recalls. "And I said, 'Well, it's not going to be *we*.'"

"'What do you mean?'"

"'Well, Mom, you gotta die first.' But I said, 'I promise, I'll make you famous.' It was funny. We laughed, you know, and then she'd think about it."

"'Well, okay, I'll go.'"

"'No,' I said, 'you don't have to die now, but I'll tell you what, Mom. At the point you're gone, the shit is gonna hit the fan.'"

In the final months, there was always a crisis, so emergencies came to seem like the normal way of things. Margaret's trach plugged up regularly; she contracted one infection after another, each weakening her further. She couldn't bear odors of any kind, so all cooking was done out in the carport. If someone walked in with perfume on, Margaret would have breathing spasms. "Mother lived for seventeen months in this state," Gayla says. "It wasn't a life. She never left her home to go outside except by ambulance."

As her physical struggles intensified, her spiritual battles subsided. Her granddaughter Jenan recalls her grandma's baptism as the turning point. Margaret had sold Avon to a retired preacher's wife; the man agreed to forgo his usual method of dunking in favor of sprinkling holy water on the dying woman's forehead. "The light in my grandma's eyes when she was baptized; she was laughing, which was something I hadn't seen in a long time," Jenan says. "Then I saw it again the night before she died. Peacefulness. I remember asking her, 'Have you been able to deal with your anger towards Grandpa?' And she was at peace with it. She had been able to work through that. It was really nice knowing that she went being able to forgive, to have peace in her heart."

By March 1996, Margaret was ready to die. Gayla says she offered to "pull one more rabbit out of a hat" and keep her going for another month or two, but Margaret declined. The day she left for the hospital, Margaret asked that her two old cats be put to sleep.

SOMEONE, NOT GAYLA, told her the cats were gone, though it was her daughter who gave her the details. There was finality in that act which transcended all the other preparations for death. In her mind's eye, she could see their funeral: David digging a hole at the river's edge for the box that held their bodies; the grandchildren with flowers for the grave, reciting the only prayer they knew, "Now I lay me down to sleep ..."; the group singing the only song everyone knew: "Happy Birthday." By the time Gayla was done telling her the story, they both were crying. Her kitties were gone. She was so tired.

It was a Monday when they all filed through to say their goodbyes. Margaret told Gayla to fight like hell: "Get the bastards," a commandment her daughter put aside for the moment. Her anger had been growing, but there was only so much room for it in her life right now. Like her sister, Gayla relished a good fight, and nothing riled her so much as injustice inflicted upon her loved ones. There would be time for this battle—just not yet.

After all the family left, Margaret slipped into a sleep so sound the nurses took it for a coma. Gayla was there when she woke, though. Margaret grabbed her daughter's hand and said, "This is tough, Gayla, so tough." Gayla held her hand and reminded her of everyone waiting for her in heaven: Perley, old friends, the cats. "Cats," Margaret whispered, smiling. She drifted off again. The next morning, she died while Eva was there holding her hand.

The Old Alley Place

Mike Power can't tell you exactly when he learned that the ranch he and his wife, Georgina, bought in 1980 had once belonged to Ed Alley, founder of the Zonolite Corporation. The Powers aren't locals: she grew up in North Dakota; he was raised in Iowa. Although Mike Power is a self-described history buff, he found the Alley connection to be merely interesting at the time they bought the place. What he does recall, vividly, is the moment that the fact became important. The news that Libby's Zonolite was laced with asbestos and had already killed at least two hundred people had just made headlines in a Seattle newspaper, and his grandchildren were visiting. "My granddaughter wanted some cinnamon for her ice cream. So I came over here," he demonstrates, opening the spice cupboard at the bottom of the staircase between the kitchen and the living room, "got this out, popped the top, and shook a little out for her." He pauses. "And it was like, 'What in the world is this?' Georgina says, 'It looks like that Zonolite stuff.' Here I'd just dumped the stuff on my granddaughter's food."

Power is a bear of a man, not tall but solid. He takes an intense interest in the world around him. Outside he shows me where a family of pileated woodpeckers nested for a few seasons. He likes animals, wild and domestic. When they first moved here, Mike and Georgina decided to do a little farming. "We were both raised on farms; we knew we wanted to live on a farm," he says. "We had horses down in Nevada, and I'd hauled five, six horses up here, I don't remember how many. We always wanted to have other things, and so when I decided to just completely quit working, we threw ourselves into the farm. We had a little dairy, pigs, chickens, pheasants, peacocks, quail, ducks, geese—Lord, we had everything. Goats, sheep—we had a little bit of everything."

Mike spent most of the first two decades they lived at the Alley place renovating the old buildings. The caretaker's cottage, he figures, was built by 1926—all the newspapers in the wall are dated

prior to that. He'd heard—and discarded—a story that the caretaker wore a wooden leg he had carved himself. When it wore out,
he would toss it under the porch and whittle a new one. Power became a believer when he excavated to pour a new foundation
under the building and found an old wooden leg. But even with
the new concrete, the gold Zonolite insulation filters out from
underneath, glittering in the dirt under lilies wilted by October's
frosts. There are different grades of Zonolite, from the one fine as
dust that ended up on the ice cream, to granules a little smaller
than peas, to flakes the size of a quarter. Alley appears to have used
it all at his little ranch, contaminating the entire place in his zeal
for discovery and invention.

A hundred feet away is a little shack that houses the pump that
supplies the Power family with water. Mike opens the wooden door
and takes a few steps down before turning to apologize. "I used to
scrub it out two or three times a year," he says. "I'm a little embar-
rassed to have you see it like this." It is perhaps 7 by 8 feet, with
an open pit in the far corner that is their well. There are cobwebs
hanging along the ceiling, glittering with Zonolite, and gold-tinted
dirt in the corners. When they bought the place, he says, there was
a wooden box filled with Zonolite at the foot of the stairs where
the former owners had stored tubers—rutabagas, carrots, and
such—during the winter. Once the news broke about asbestos in
the Zonolite, Power stopped his housekeeping. The Environmental Protection Agency has given him no opinion on the safety of
the water in the open pit.

He also stopped his remodeling. Mike was turning half of an old
barn into a bunkhouse for guests. "I just laid my tools down and
walked away." He scrapes at the chinking to show me how good it
is—pliable after so many years and laced with the telltale gold
flecks. "Now there are people who are so desperate and so afraid
that the only thing they have is their home, and they expect to sell
it in their old age and, frankly, eat it. That's the way at our place,
you know? That's what we have to look forward to in our future.
Eat that thing in the future, have to sell it at some point, and what
we get out of that is going to keep us in our old age.

"If it's worthless, you're in trouble. Or if they come in and clean all the buildings off of it, and you have a bare piece of land, it's a lot different matter."

The main house, Power tells me, was built around the turn of the century. The square, two-story structure is made from hand-hewn logs. Mike and his wife took great care in restoring it, matching the molding around the windows and doors as closely as possible to the original. As Power shows me around his house, two things become clear: his wife is a fine housekeeper, and still the soft gold dust sifts out everywhere. Power is wheezing a bit after we climb the short but steep and narrow staircase to the bedrooms on the second floor. He has been diagnosed with asbestosis, but so far the rest of his family has not. He didn't get around to remodeling the upstairs, and explains that they are hesitant to tear out the old carpet for fear of the dust it would raise. The Zonolite is in their bedroom, a few days' worth accumulating on the ledge in their closet. He opens the door to a little girl's room, the bed unmade as if she had slept in it the night before. Another doorway leads to his grandson's bedroom. "The EPA found an original burlap bag of the Zonolite in the attic, right in that corner," he points above the twin bed. "They wanted to know what I wanted done with it, and I said just leave it there."

His grandchildren no longer spend the night. "The kids like bringing their kids out here, they like to be out here. But we've asked them not to stay here anymore."

TWO

Almost Paradise

To approach Libby from the south or east is to enter a foreign country, with the landscape reflecting the culture as it changes. Montana Highway 2 stretches across the state's northern Hi-Line through buffalo and antelope country, Plains Indian country, crossing the seemingly endless expansive prairie that gives the Big Sky Country its name, before ending abruptly where the Rocky Mountains begin, on the western edge of the Blackfeet Reservation at Glacier National Park. Trees close in as the route continues west from the town of Kalispell along a precarious two-lane mountain road, bisecting small wet meadows where one is likely to see moose, elk, and bear at dawn and dusk, before topping out in a narrow river valley: home of the Libby Loggers, high school teams named for the region's primary industry; the Kootenai River Falls, scene of the Meryl Streep film *The River Wild*; and 17 miles upstream from town, the river tamed: Lake Koocanusa, where the Kootenai was dammed during a construction project that flooded the local economy with jobs during the 1960s.

From the south, one can avoid the Flathead Valley's incessant tourist traffic, drawn by Glacier National Park, the ski resort in Whitefish, and the boating culture of Flathead Lake (prior to being dammed, the largest natural freshwater lake in the western United States), by turning onto Highway 200 and following the meanders of the Flathead River to its junction with William Clark's fork of the mighty Columbia. Traffic is sparse. The treeless hills are undeveloped with the exception of a handful of small towns barely large enough to warrant a post office. Late autumn shadows hold the warmth of the sun that casts them, reflected off the gold and yellow aspen, cottonwood, and larch. It's not unusual to see bald eagles and osprey fishing the broad waters. When the river flattens and stretches into the reservoir that is part of the vast dammed-up Pend Oreille lake system, lifestyle and landscape collide. It's spinning rod culture, bait shops and Rainier beer, motorboats and RV parks, a region of former rivers that gives locals more in common with their neighbors in eastern Washington and northern Idaho than with the rest of Montana.

The association is not an entirely flattering one. The region is well-known to human rights activists across the United States, who "refer to this whole area—northwestern Montana, eastern Washington, and the Idaho panhandle—as the Nazi Corridor," says Ken Toole of the Montana Human Rights Network. "These groups are very prevalent in this part of the country." That's not to say Libby is full of armed Aryan brothers. Although neighboring towns like Thompson Falls, Montana, and Hayden Lake, Idaho, are home to the Militia of Montana and Aryan Nations, until the asbestos issue brought the EPA to town, Libby residents pretty much stuck to a moderate distrust of the government and knee-jerk intolerance for environmentalism—the reaction of a de facto company town to declines in the logging and mining industries.

Historian Dave Walter says this cultural affiliation is based more on a feeling he gets than on anything else, though when pushed for evidence he attributes it to isolation, a function of geography and weather. "It's easier to get out to Spokane [Washington] and Coeur d'Alene [Idaho] than Missoula most of the year. It's not only where the highways are, but the quality of them," he says. "I had to spend a week up there one winter, and I thought I'd died and gone to hell. I'd never seen so much snow in my life." Walter, a researcher for the state historical society, notes that Lincoln County residents refer to themselves as being "at the end of the driveway" that starts in Kalispell. Libby's isolation from the rest of Montana "dictates where they might shop, where they might vacation, where they might fish. And media stuff—they get mostly Spokane television, so that's all the north Idaho news with a little dab of western Montana news," he says. "Look at what teams Libby plays out of the conference: they schedule Idaho, eastern Washington, or Canada. That's a giveaway."

Libby lies in what was the last corner of the state to be settled, and even though the railroad sent a line through in 1892, winter's endless snowfall kept the town relatively isolated for about half of every year. Libby's reaction was to find security in insularity. The pre-1900 settlers formed the Pioneer Society, and for decades these old families ran the town. People who moved in after the turn of the century say they found it hard to fit in. There were few industries that provided steady jobs—a relative concept that included seasonal logging for the local lumber mill—so Libby residents defended these businesses as though their lives depended on it, which in a large sense they did.

There were newcomers who stayed, attracted by Libby's natural beauty and the pace of small-town life. There is no wrong side of the tracks, river, or highway. Virtually the only crimes are domestic, and for those who love the outdoors the mountains and rivers do not care how long one has been in residence. The population of Lincoln County grew steadily and unremarkably from 3,638 in 1910, to a peak of 18,063 in 1970 during the Libby Dam construction, back down to about 12,000 today.

Les Skramstad was one who settled in and one of hundreds, possibly thousands, who will pay for that choice with his life. He came for a short visit in 1954 and found half a century later that he'd made a life, raised a family, here. A writer for a New York–based men's magazine described Les in a 2001 article on the asbestos tragedy as grizzled and bowlegged. In fact, while he carries his small frame on legs that speak loudly of his cowboy days, his beard is nearly always well trimmed, and whenever he goes out he dresses for town. As he talks of his youth, his voice now whispered and hoarse with the effects of the asbestos scars wrapped around his lungs, there's a glint in his sixty-five-year-old eyes that brings out the handsome young man torn between his wanderlust and his responsibilities at home.

"We were just typical young people," he says. "Thought we were going to live forever and had a good time while we's doing it."

Les recalls the 1950s as a time of freedom in his life. A young man could support himself just fine by hiring on day jobs, so long as he didn't need too much. That life suited Les. He was born in North Dakota, but moved around with his sharecropper parents. The family lived as well in Wyoming and Washington, where Les picked up work on ranches, as a Forest Service firefighter, a Bureau of Reclamation surveyor, and as a nanny and maid at a Yellowstone-area tourist lodge before he turned eighteen. He drove to Libby to visit some friends in March 1954 and ended up stranded. "I didn't plan on staying more than a week. But anyway, things happen," he says. "It turned 14 below zero the first night that I was here and cracked the block in my car, so I was stuck here." It was close to springtime in Libby, still winter out on the plains, so Les settled in for a while, picking up a job with the Forest Service 65 miles north in Rexburg. He went to work on Monday, came back Friday. His weekends, he says, were spent chasing girls.

One day he was driving along and saw two pretty young women, Norita Gardiner and Rose McQueen, walking down the road. "I drove up alongside of them and asked if they wanted a lift. This was kind of the way you picked up girls. And naturally they said no," he says. "But I didn't take that for an absolute concrete answer, so I kept following along. 'I'll take you home, take you out, whatever you want to do.'" They talked some more, and a few days later when he again offered a ride, the girls said yes. Just before Christmas 1955, Norita said yes to marriage.

"Les was a very handsome young man," Norita says by way of explanation. She's quick to smile, her affection for her husband slipping out in a schoolgirl's laugh. "I liked the western clothes, I liked the boots, the hat. He always dressed nice. Still does today. He likes white shirts, always wears a cowboy hat, always wears jeans, boots. He was always polite, but not overly. He wasn't one of those real rowdy types. I wasn't either. Suited me just fine; still does, forty-six years later."

When they first married, Norita had a job keeping the books at the local bank. Les started out supporting them by working for the local lumber mill, run by the Neils family, as a pole roller and a forklift driver, but he wasn't ready to settle down. "I was sick of working at the sawmill," he says. "Neils were really decent people, but I always wanted to be a cowboy." Les and Norita came from plains people—although Les would put in his time as a logger, they weren't born to the woods. "By God, when I first came to Libby, I came out of the prairies, the Dakotas; I didn't even know the country," Norita says. "I couldn't believe all the trees in this country. And all the loggers." By 1957, they had a baby girl named Laurel. Now with a family, Norita quit her job to take care of their daughter, and Les realized his time to fool around was limited. "I thought, if I'm going to do this, I better do it now. So I took to the road, and sent her back to her mother in South Dakota." It might have been a good life had Les been a more typical cowboy, finding his soul's peace and satisfaction in the job's hard work and solitude, and had he been single. But cowboy wages didn't go far, and Les concedes it was no way to raise a family.

From eastern Montana he lit out for Kentucky, planning to work at a racehorse farm. California was next, but after a few months of scraping by and sleeping in his car, Les gave up—temporarily in his mind—and headed back to Libby to visit his folks, who had moved to town with his encouragement. He rested up a few days, eating better than he had in a long time, then announced he was heading back to California.

"Finally Ma says, 'Well, I got a surprise for you.' That was the last thing I needed was another surprise. She says, 'Norita and Laurel are here.' I said, 'How in the hell did they get here?' I knew she didn't have any money." It turned out that Norita's brother lived in Libby, and when his wife had a stroke, they asked Norita to come back and help take care of their two kids. Les wasn't going anywhere.

There wasn't much to do in Libby in those days, the Skramstads say. They mostly palled around with friends, with outsiders who had trouble making it within the town's establishment, going dancing in Idaho, going to Kalispell for coffee, or just going, driving around the countryside in the middle of the night, stopping so one friend could fulfill his ambition to run barefoot across a meadow. Once, on a lark, Les and a friend bought a car for $40. "We all got on top of it and smashed the top in, filled it up with dirt, ran it down Main Street of Libby," Norita says. "The dirt was just flying."

Norita recalls these times as sweet for being so mundane. This is when she first became acquainted with Gayla Vatland, a little blonde fireball who lived with her parents across the highway from the Skramstads. The beginnings of their acquaintance were innocuous enough: music drew the two immigrant families from the plains together. Perley was a real musician and could play anything, so Les was always across the street, learning, picking along. By that time, Eva had married and moved away, but Gayla still lived at home. "She was just this little gal. I'd see her on the street. She'd say, 'Hello, Mrs. Skramstad.' I was nineteen years old, so that sounded pretty old," Norita says with a laugh. "I'd say, 'Les, what's that girl's name?' I'd forget it. Next time she'd go by, 'Mrs. Skramstad.' What's that girl's name? *Gayla.* So we had a baby, we named her Gayla."

In the aftermath of the asbestos plague, Gayla says she has learned much about human nature. "It isn't a matter of finding out who your friends and your enemies are. It's about finding out what people are really made of," she says. Her old friends the Skramstads, she says, turned out to be the finest kind of people, and Les her greatest ally.

LIBBY WAS, and many claim still is, a place where a person can scrape by without many resources. Les picked up jobs at the sawmill, doing construction on a dam being built at the nearest town, Troy, 15 miles to the west. He cut his own firewood, hunted deer, and fished local creeks to feed his new family. They got by on unemployment during the winter of 1957, stretching $32 a week to cover rent and bills, with about $10 left over each month for food. It was the hardest season of their married life. Les found work as an auto mechanic in Kalispell for a while, but finally had to swallow his pride and go back to the sawmill, a job he dreaded, after Norita had another baby. When the chance came to get temporary work at the vermiculite mine, he weighed the choice heavily.

"I'd heard around here, if you could get a job at Zonolite, at the mine there, you were set for life," he says. But when he went down to ask about the job, the boss said it would only last a month, until the end of September. That would set Les up for another winter of living on unemployment. "I said I don't think I can do it and walked back out the door. And I got to my car and I thought, 'Geez, I want that job.' I was relying solely on my ambition and my abilities, which were pretty dang good in those days. Feller thinks he's 10 foot tall and bulletproof when you're that age. I was twenty-three and I thought, 'Boy, if I can't make it here, I'll scrape by some way.'"

So he walked back in and took the job, then faced the prospect of telling his young wife what he had done. "She was not happy. She remembered '57 and I do too. That's a real lasting thing in my memory. But anyway, 7 o'clock that morning I went to work for Zonolite."

THE REGION SURROUNDING THE small town of Libby is an anomaly in Montana. Enveloped by rich cedar and conifer forests, the landscape is eerily dank and dense compared with the open, windy country that characterizes the rest of the state. Even locals sometimes describe their surroundings as claustrophobic. But the humidity of the Pacific rain shadow has also made Libby a bustling logging town for most of the last century; the climate is relatively favorable for tree-growing, though it was the promise of minerals under those trees that initially drew prospectors to the area in the mid-1800s. Many had used up their luck elsewhere and ended up in this farthest northwestern corner of Montana as a last resort. While a few got lucky, the gold fever of these early miners rarely panned out. It took a second mining boom starting in 1885, along with the railroad coming through in 1892, to populate the region for good. This time prospectors eked out a modest existence on the proceeds of silver, lead, coal, and a smattering of gold. The economy stabilized a bit when Wisconsin timber magnate Julius Neils took over the sawmill, but even that work was seasonal.

The townspeople, however, saw themselves as blessed. The newspaper of those days is full of stories of gay skating parties, happy youth playing basketball tournaments with kids from neighboring towns, a lively intellectual community nurtured by regular Chautauqua lectures brought in by the local Women's Club. There

was an occasional bar shooting or problems with bootleggers setting up stills in the region's creeks or running whiskey from
Canada. But it was quaint, harmless stuff of the sort expected in a
rough-and-tumble Wild West town. The overwhelming image is of
a community in love with itself, full of hardworking white men and
their families acting out one of the last scenes in the greater Manifest Destiny drama on Montana's final frontier.

It wasn't until the 1920s that Libby's second source of economic
wealth was realized: vermiculite. Literally a mountain of it lay
about 7 miles northeast of town as the raven flies. The ore deposit
first caught the attention of Libby businessman Edward Alley during World War I, when the federal government was looking for
vanadium as a source material for steel. A few oral and historical
reports describe a local politician named Henry Brink showing
samples of a "rotten mica"–like substance to his friend Alley, who
then acquired (some say underhandedly) the mineral claim from
which it came. Other accounts describe Alley poking around old
mines on the mountain and accidentally setting the flame of his
candle to some vermiculite ore in a tunnel wall, which popped and
sizzled and expanded before his curious eyes.

A 1928 U.S. Geological Survey report characterizes the deposit
as topping off the Algonkian Belt series, rock laid down prior to
the Cambrian period about four or five billion years ago. Geologists have dated the vermiculite and asbestos deposits at approximately 100 million years of age. The USGS surveyors describe
dikes of "amphibole asbestos" up to 14 feet wide jutting through
the rock. "In several places this substance composes from 50 to 75
percent of the country rock," they write. "A small amount has
been mined for experimental purposes, but no commercial product is reported." The vermiculite is what really had caught their
attention. The deposit was the largest known in the world: at least
100 feet wide, 1,000 feet long, and deeper than they could determine. "The most striking features of the vermiculite from Rainy
Creek are its properties of expanding enormously when heated and
at the same time assuming golden or silvery lusters. The expanded
material floats on water and is nearly as light as a cork. It appears

to have a very low heat conductivity and to be capable of resisting high temperature. These qualities at once suggest it to be useful for heat and cold insulation and similar purposes."

By the time of his death in 1935, Alley had turned the curious mineral into an industry that would help support Libby nearly to the next century. But to start with, he was just a small-time entrepreneur with the soul of an inventor. His attitude gave him something in common with the state's indigenous people. Historian Joseph Kinsey Howard wrote in his classic book, *Montana: High, Wide and Handsome*, that the region's Indians lived as if all native plants had worth—if something seemed useless, it was only because they had not discovered its purpose. Alley looked at his mountain of rotten mica in much the same way: there was so much of it, there had to be some use for it. He hauled samples down to his home, a pretty little ranch on the north side of the Kootenai River, and began experimenting. The ore was layered, paper-thin sheets that held water. When heated, the water turned to steam and popped the layers out. Alley built a furnace out of rock and clay on a slope so he could pour vermiculite in the top and catch the expanded rock—now light as popcorn—where it came out at the bottom. He tinkered with the temperature, firing up with waste from the sawmill, searching for the perfect balance of heat and timing. Eventually he discarded the cast-iron floor as too frail to withstand the heat, replacing it with bricks. With this setup he could turn out 4 tons of expanded vermiculite a day. He named his invention Zonolite, and used it to insulate all his own buildings, such that nearly eighty years later it still spills out, fine as silt, from loose baseboards and cracks in the walls and ceilings.

By 1924 the local paper touted Zonolite as having "a hundred and one uses." The list grew nearly as fast as Alley and, later, his team of researchers could brainstorm. Zonolite provided insulation against the cold and heat; it was easy to install and marketed as a do-it-yourself product for residential housing. It could be used in wall plaster and wallpaper, as a paint additive, as bronze printer's ink, and when mixed with plastic, in place of drywall. A Billings, Montana, company began to build floor tiling and lightweight,

weatherproof roofs out of the material. Hollywood lauded Zonolite
as ideal for soundproofing movie studios and enhancing theater
acoustics. A fruit shipping firm announced it could save $30,000
a year per ship by insulating with Zonolite. In later years locals
even came up with recipes to use a fine, powdery form of Zonolite
for making bread and cookies in the hope of creating baked goods
resistant to mold:

Whole Wheat Zonobread

Two pkg. dry yeast in ½ cup warm water and three cups
    whole wheat flour
1-½ cups of water and three cups No. 4 Vermiculite
    Feed Grade
1 tsp. salt
¼ cup white flour
⅓ cup molasses
¼ cup sugar

At first the orders came for a carload at a time, a ton here, a
couple of tons there. The first shipment by "large automobile car"
was sent to a company in Hillsboro, Ohio, that manufactured
office safes, bank vaults, and steel filing cabinets. The timing was
good. Though some modern proponents of the mining industry
would argue that there is still plenty of wealth to dig up in the area,
the region's gold and silver deposits had turned out to be rather
modest, and the fur trade had long been trapped out. The town's
only sizable commerce before Alley's enterprise gained momentum
was J. Neils's family-owned sawmill. By the mid-1920s, small shipments of Zonolite were going all over the country and beyond:
Wisconsin, Nebraska, Missouri, and New Jersey, with more inquiries coming from Scotland, Japan, and London. A couple of
California businessmen promised to export Zonolite to Mexico.
Alley spent his spare time traveling back east, begging for invest-
ment capital to support his vision.

    There were obstacles to building a world-class industry in a re-
mote corner of Montana, and in a 1926 interview with the *Flathead*

Monitor newspaper, Alley says he nearly went broke doing it. "Before Zonolite was securely established I had disposed of everything I had except a ranch and this had been mortgaged." To begin with, Alley had competitors. He didn't own the mountain, but only some of the mineral claims on it. Other miners started up their own vermiculite businesses, including the Vermiculite and Asbestos Co., the Kootenai Valley Products Co., and the Black Mica and Micalite Companies. The railroad had a virtual monopoly on transportation and could hold the region's businesses hostage with high freight rates if it chose to. But Alley had some important allies. He and Libby's mayor, Murray Gay, were from the same hometown of Wilbur, Nebraska, and shared family and business matters. They were married to sisters, and in 1923 Alley sold Gay his interest in the swank Libby Hotel (hot and cold running water "in practically every room" and the only first-class restaurant between Spokane and Kalispell). So when Alley decided to incorporate the Zonolite Company in 1927, he naturally brought in his brother-in-law as partner. Gay served as secretary-treasurer, a role he would fill until his death in 1946.

Alley also had pull at the town's daily newspaper. While some of the other fledgling companies on the mountain received occasional mentions in the *Western News*, Alley's efforts command the big headlines. When he bemoans the fact that high railroad freight costs may slow the growth of his business, a reporter immediately jumps in to avow that "if a suitable freight rate is granted, this industry will develop into very large proportions in the very near future." Three months later, the paper proclaims the "welcome news" that the Great Northern Railroad has reduced its shipping rates from $17.50 to $17 a ton for Zonolite headed to the East Coast.

Alley also persuaded the town's Commercial Club in 1925 to endorse *his* operation over the other mining companies, the club promising "to do whatever it can to assist in any further needed financing of the enterprise." As the other mines on Vermiculite Mountain merged or collapsed, competition narrowed down to two: Alley's Zonolite Company and Bill Hillis's Universal Insulation

Company. The two men were reported to be "bitter enemies," and both carried a gun when they went to their respective claims in case they saw the other. Old-timer Bob Holiday, who owned a dump truck and worked for both men, said the rivalry yielded interesting results. "The Zonolite had the best ore," Holiday recalled prior to his death in 1997. "They just drove trucks into the pit and shoveled trucks full by hand. ... On the north side, the ore was not clean, so [Universal Insulation] had to devise methods of cleaning the ore. Many methods were tried and patented. When Zonolite used all of their pure ore, they started trying methods of cleaning the ore. Every method they tried the Universal Insulation had patented.

"That may have been expensive to clear up," Holiday noted wryly. Before Alley died of a brief illness just shy of his fifty-seventh birthday in 1935, he sold the Zonolite Company to "Detroit interests," which were fronted by a man named William B. Mayo, chief engineer for the Ford Motor Company. Hillis, meanwhile, sold out to a cadre of "Chicago capitalists" whose members included Phillip and Lester Armour, of the Armour Meat Packing company. In 1939 the two former rivals merged under the name Universal Zonolite Insulation Company, referred to by locals simply as Zonolite. That's when things really started to take off.

As in Alley's day, the challenge was less to dig out and process vermiculite than to find buyers and ship it out. It was cheaper, Zonolite directors had learned, to ship the smaller, unprocessed rock than to pay for a railcar of expanded airy vermiculite. So they opened up processing plants in Minnesota, Chicago, Kansas City, Detroit, Pennsylvania, Hawaii, New York, and South Carolina, adding Cuba, Puerto Rico, India, Australia, Pakistan, Venezuela, Chile, Brazil, and Italy on the international scene. Eventually nearly three hundred such plants processed Libby ore. As of 1941, most of the vermiculite was destined to serve as "house fill," loose insulation that could be poured in between the walls. During the next decade, Zonolite gained popularity as a concrete mixer and additive for plaster. Libby vermiculite served as the "aggregate" or base material for 20 percent of the plaster manufactured in the

entire country in 1949. Sales nearly doubled that year to almost
$4.2 million, according to a report in *The Western News*, largely be-
cause of the growing popularity of Terra-lite, a soil additive much
like the vermiculite potting soil still used by gardeners today.

In short, Libby's vermiculite went everywhere.

UNLIKE MOST MEN WHO worked for Zonolite, Earl Lovick had
never held a grunt's job. Yet Libby knew Earl. He was the black-
smith's son, the six-year-old boy sent to live with his mother's
people in Winnipeg after his dad died. He was the young man with
a college degree who came back to Libby after a stint in the army
(serving in North Africa and Italy during World War II) and took
the accountant's job in 1948. He progressed through the ranks,
steady as they come: assistant manager, general manager, and manager of administration, staying on after Zonolite was sold to the
multinational W.R. Grace & Company in 1963. During his four
decades at the mine, he became Citizen Earl, serving on the hospital and bank boards; presiding over the Lions Club, Chamber of
Commerce, and school board; counting the town's newspaper editor, money men, and politicians among his friends. He could open
any door with a phone call and must have wielded his power judi-
ciously: by all accounts, the man was well liked. When Zonolite
started leasing a piece of land by the river to the Little League for
$1 a year, Lovick was chosen to hit the first pitch at the ball field's
dedication. In 1964 the local Jaycees named him "Boss of the
Year." After he retired in 1983, Lovick continued to act as a paid
consultant to the company. To Libby he was the face of Grace.

But when Earl died in 1998, he left behind a few close friends
who prefer not to talk about him with strangers, others who will say
only that Earl was popular. His widow, his second wife, Bonnie, has
so far shunned the media—which could have something to do with
the fact that asbestos plaintiffs started naming her husband's estate
as a defendant in Earl's absence. And then there are those—lots of
people—who thought they knew Earl, who now say while shaking
their heads, "He seemed like a good man." Because the truth is,
Earl Lovick knew that Zonolite was laced with asbestos, that Alley's

miracle ore was killing miners and maybe even other townspeople.
And he did nothing to warn them.

From the beginning, mining Zonolite was an experiment. Nearly
all the equipment, machinery, and processes had to be designed
from scratch or borrowed from other industries and modified. By
the time Lovick took the assistant manager's position in 1954, the
process was pretty well set in place. The men strip-mined, digging
around on the surface of the mountain from the bottom up, eventually lowering the elevation on the 400-acre site by 100 feet. They
used huge power shovels to carve out steep stairlike benches,
28 feet tall, into the side of the hill. Big Euclid dump trucks, called
"Eucs," could handle three shovel loads of rock per trip, dumping
waste into Carney Creek and ore onto a conveyor belt at the transfer point. From there, rock, vermiculite, asbestos, and all were con-
veyed to a series of silos, separated by grade. The ore was run
through a wet mill, a dry mill, then trucked down either to a storage
facility on the bank of the Kootenai River, where raw vermiculite
was loaded onto railcars and shipped elsewhere for processing, or
to the expanding plant in town next to the baseball fields, where
Zonolite employees ran it through a furnace, popping it up to full
size, and bagged it for shipping.

Men worked at all of these points: greasing conveyor belt rollers,
opening gates, cleaning, bagging, loading. Nearly all of it was dusty
work, Earl Lovick testified during a deposition for Les Skramstad's
case against Grace. And all the dust, he admitted under pointed
questioning, contained asbestos.

Lovick knew more about asbestos than the average person in
1959, the year Les was hired on. As part of Zonolite's management team he had access to inspection reports filed by the State
of Montana that warned about high levels of asbestos in the dust
at the mine. He'd read precise descriptions in these reports of the
damage that would be done to a man's lungs by asbestos, and
statements that those simply living near an asbestos mine could
suffer respiratory damage. He knew that the form of asbestos at
Zonolite's mine was called "tremolite," that it was a straighter
fiber than commercial forms of asbestos. He knew, point by point,

the places in Zonolite's operation that leaked tremolite asbestos dust. And he knew that more than a third of the mine's employees were having lung problems.

Lovick testified that he believed the workers who had abnormal lung X rays must have come to the company in that condition. Local doctors—one surgeon, the rest general practitioners, none with pulmonary expertise—could not conclusively link lung problems at the mine to the asbestos, and Lovick took their word as authoritative. The miners were provided with respirators, and they should have worn them. "We believed if they wore the respirators they would be breathing air which was within the allowable concentration range," he testified in 1997. Earlier, when lawyers asked him if he or anyone else at Zonolite had told the workers exactly why wearing respirators was so important, he said no. "There are some things that [there] shouldn't be a need to explain. You shouldn't have to tell an employee that they shouldn't put their fingers to a piece of red hot iron, either, but we never told them that." This applied, too, to the kids who were caught playing in the waste vermiculite piles by the baseball fields. "We were not successful in keeping them away," Lovick said, his unspoken conclusion being that if people didn't do what they were told, they brought misfortune upon themselves.

As for the studies showing that asbestos could be harmful to people living nearby, Lovick claimed he neither worried about nor warned Libby residents because those reports dealt with commercial asbestos facilities, not vermiculite mines with asbestos contamination. When Grace purchased Zonolite in 1963, Lovick retained his job, as did all the managers at the mine. In retrospect Lovick insisted that Zonolite managers did everything practical to follow measures recommended by the state inspector for cleaning up the company's dust problem, before and after the change in ownership. They oiled the road to keep dust down, tested and rejected a vacuum cleaner system, installed new fans, tried to keep the milling equipment well maintained, and instigated a monthly "sweepdown" of the dry mill.

Lovick served on a safety committee formed by Zonolite, which included both management and workers. "[They] would do an inspection each month of the operations, and anything that they deemed to be unsafe they would record and turn into management for correction, if possible," he said. That did not include, however, the fact that there was asbestos in the dust. Until Grace managers began to leak out the word "tremolite" in the late 1970s, no one on record said anything about asbestos to the employees. According to Lovick, they simply should have known. "There's every reason to think these employees were aware of it," he said. "Among other things, the union, which they all belonged to, had information on the hazards of asbestos to their welfare." But in fact, one of the mine's last two living union representatives, a feisty old man named Bob Wilkins, says he didn't find out until 1979, when he got the news from a federal health inspector and then confronted Lovick. By then, although he had told everyone who would listen, it was too late for most of the men.

AS A THEOLOGIAN, Lutheran pastor Les Nelson has considered the question of evil in the world. It is not an idle exercise for him: Nelson's congregation includes, for instance, an extended family of forty members, thirty of whom have been diagnosed with asbestos-related diseases from the mine on Vermiculite Mountain. He doesn't name Lovick directly, speaking instead of the pressures on Grace's middlemen, managers with families, needing to keep their jobs, working under pressure first from Zonolite officials in Chicago, later from W.R. Grace executives on the East Coast, to do their jobs well and to fix the dust problem without spending too much money. It is a tad uncomfortable to see things from Lovick's point of view: the shades of gray lead Nelson and me to consider as reasonable convenient ways to minimize the asbestos problem until hundreds are dying. Would it take someone extraordinary to do things differently?

Despite what he knew about asbestos and disease at the mine, about the real threat to his fellow townspeople, Earl Lovick never warned his neighbors. Maybe he was a bad man, or maybe the scope of the impending tragedy was simply too large to accept and he lied to himself as well as everyone else. After all, Lovick had

raised his kids here too. And he never left Libby: the man who believed his children never played in the vermiculite piles because
he had told them not to died of cancer in 1998.

ON HIS FIRST DAY AT Zonolite in 1959, Les Skramstad was sent
to work in the six-story dry mill, where a series of screens and
shakers separated out the valuable vermiculite ore from the rocks
and debris that comprise a mountain. "Unfortunately, virtually
every one of us who worked there, their first job was in the dry
mill," Les says. "Probably that's the worst place you could ever
imagine being. If they had hundreds of vacuum cleaners blowing
all the dirt in town in this room, that might be comparable. You
started out sweeping. There were beams running all over, and
equipment, shakers and screens and such. Your job was to sweep
and clean that because that dust stuck to everything. It would stick
to a wire, stand up that tall," he says, spreading his thumb and
forefinger about an inch and a half apart, "and stick to a lightbulb.
You couldn't see the lightbulbs. Anyway, your job was to sweep
that down on the floor. All the time you were sweeping, it was boil-
ing like that because it wanted to get airborne. Then there was
holes in the floor every once in a while and you'd sweep through
the holes. And when you swept it through the holes, you can imagine what it was like down on the next floor.

"When you got it all down there, as much as you could get,
you'd get on an elevator and go down to the next floor and start
the whole thing over again. When we'd get it all down to the last
floor, it would be 3 feet deep. Then we'd take a wheelbarrow and
carry it over to the waste belt, and that carried it on over the side
of the mountain and just puked it over the edge."

The men who worked in the dry mill were given respirators to
wear—masks designed to cover their mouths and noses. Many
complained that they clogged up almost immediately in the dusty
conditions, and discarded this protection as useless. Others report
that the masks never sealed quite tight, and even those who did
wear them had streaks of dust underneath their noses within minutes. But the dry mill was for short-timers. Les was out of there

within a couple of days. For the next three weeks he worked as a skip-drag operator on the small railcars that hauled ore from the dry mill to storage bins, and eyed the calendar nervously as his month came to an end. One day the company put up a notice that it was hiring a dump boss. "Well, I hadn't the foggiest notion what that was either, but that didn't matter," Les says. It was a "bid" job, a union position. "If I got a bid job, then I was pretty sure I was going to stay at least the winter. So I put my bid in right then." As it turned out, the dump boss job took him out of the dust and put him out on the side of the mountain, overseeing the big Euclid dump trucks as they chucked waste rock over the side of a ravine into Carney Creek. Les took over for the Euc drivers when they needed a coffee break, and says he would have stayed in that job forever except for an accident one December afternoon.

"This particular day it snowed a little and rained a little, and it was just a typical nasty day. We had [tire] chains on, huge ones," he says. The shift was nearly over when his friend, twenty-seven-year-old Gordon Torkelson, decided he'd had enough wrestling with the big Euc, made even more awkward by the tire chains. "He said, 'I'm taking these damn chains off. I've had it, I can't stand another minute of it.' And I said, 'God, Torgie, why don't you leave 'em on? We've only got another load or two. And night shift's probably going to have to put them right back on.'

"'I don't care, they can put them back on,' he says. 'I'm taking them off.' And he's already taken one side off. I went over and took the other side off. He jumped in the cab and drove ahead, and I took the chains up. Just a few minutes, here comes Dale Smith, a Euc skinner. He didn't have a load on. I thought, 'What in the heck's going on?' And he opened the door and he said, 'Torgie just went over the bank.' God, I jumped in the cab there with him and we went up to there ... and he didn't go over the bank. He had jumped out and the Euc ran over him. Squashed him flat. Everything on him was flat. I can see that in my mind right now. ... I had just talked to him minutes ago. And there he was laying there dead, squashed. And I really did not know what I was going to do. That's an experience; I guess you have to be there in order to understand what it was really all about. It kept running through my mind, 'That could be you.'"

Torgie was the fifth man to die accidentally at Zonolite in nine years, so Les considered his options. He had a friend, Bob Cohenour, the boss at the expansion plant in town, who kept trying to entice Les to leave the hill and come work inside. After Torgie's death, Les lost his taste for the dump boss job and gave his friend a call. By then Les and Norita were expecting their third baby—the daughter they'd name after Gayla—and the pay raise that came with the job change was more than welcome. And it being winter, Les didn't mind the move inside too much either.

The team Les joined included his friend Bob and an engineer named Dave Robinson. In addition to running raw ore through the furnace, the three were charged with finding new ways to process the vermiculite, to use and market the ore. Les loved the challenge. "It was a good job. Boy I tell you, I liked that job. Bob taught me so many things that I've used through my life, such as welding, cutting metal with acetylene torches, and things like that, and figuring out how to build things.

"The experiments, you know, we were always trying to find another use for the product because there was so much of it. The whole mountain—I don't know, it might go all the way to China. And I'll sit there and tell you I thought it was a good idea because I thought it was a good product. We used it for insulating houses, we used it for making plaster. I was just on cloud nine every day. Most guys hate to go to work in the morning. I didn't. 'Cause I knew that pretty often we were going to tackle another situation, see if we could build something, make some kind of a product."

One day the trio began what Les calls "the asbestos project." Dave came down to the plant and ordered Les and Bob to take a pickup truck up the hill and bring back a load of asbestos. They drove off with a half-ton Dodge and went to see one of Les's former bosses, Orville Thorn. Thorny directed the pair up to one of the ledges dug out of the hillside, where they found an odd seam in the rock. "Over on that particular area, there was a bunch of springs, and it was a sorta grayish sort of tint. It was so pure, it was almost soft. Kinda like soap." They went at the seam with a pick and a shovel, but it was easy digging. Back down at the plant, they spread the damp material out on paper on the floor and set up heaters and fans to dry it out. "It dried really slow. Asbestos holds moisture. And there was vermiculite in it, of course, and some rock. Our job was to pick all those rocks out, all the vermiculite, and get pure asbestos with nothing else in it, not even a speck. Robinson kept on emphasizing that. 'We've got to have this 100 percent pure.'

"It took us two weeks to do that pickup load. And we were down on our hands and knees because when it started getting dry, we couldn't run the fans anymore. We could run electric heaters provided they didn't put out too much air. That was the stuff we was trying to save. I mean to tell you we were diligent in our work." They stored the asbestos in garbage cans at first. The other guys at the plant would come in and tease, "You guys still playing with this stuff?" Les says they'd stick their arms in the barrels and come out looking like they were covered with white feathers. "We'd tell them, 'Don't do that! That took us weeks!' But it was crazy stuff. We'd have these 30-gallon garbage cans that wouldn't weigh nothing. You could just stick your hand in there right to the bottom with no effort. Then we sacked that up in these bags, sewed 'em shut. And then I think Bob went up to the office and got some papers, where it was supposed to be sent to. I didn't pay no attention to it, you know. ... I think we had about twenty bags, at least twenty. We put them in the pickup, Bob took them downtown. For the life of me I can't remember if they were sent up here on the rail or on trucks. But anyway they were gone. Then we had to clean up our residue, so to speak, 'cause we had another expansion job to do. That residue, there was a lot of that asbestos.

"Looking back, I hadn't the slightest idea what we were doing," he says. "[But] it was a good place to work." He lists the benefits in a voice made hoarse by the disease that likely will kill him sometime in the next few years: they received vacation time; miners were able to buy appliances through the company at Zonolite's cost; the bosses were human and would sit and drink coffee with the men, call them by name. "I really thought the world of them. There was nothing I wouldn't have done for them. Except I don't think I would have given my life. I certainly wouldn't have given the lives of my family."

Les came home each night to a happy family. His two oldest children would rush to hang on his legs; he and Norita would greet each other with a big kiss. He would then pull off his dusty work clothes, which, thanks to a personal loan from the local bank president, Norita was able to wash in an electric-powered wringer washer. Some of the asbestos-laden dust came out in the wash, a gray sludge lying in the bottom of the tub. In the winter, she'd hang Les's wet clothes in the family living room, and as they dried, more dust would fall out. The "dirt," as she called it, was a constant, but the miners' wives simply accepted it as part of their housework.

Les says he probably would have stayed at Zonolite forever, but Norita was having trouble settling into Libby. Though the town had barely been settled a hundred years before, the first families on the scene were snobbish, she says, and newcomers like the Skramstads were treated as outcasts. "It was a real clannish town," she says. "Still is." Furthermore, to a woman raised in the great open Dakota country, the landscape of the Northwest was too close for comfort. "She gets the feeling that she's hemmed in here, which you are," Les says. In 1961, the couple decided to pull up stakes and move back to Kalispell, where they stayed for the next six years.

Les and Norita ended up with five children—three girls and two boys—and actually raised a few other kids as well. "One year Brent brought home some kid that stayed with us, what, a year?" Norita says, asking Les to refresh her memory. "And then Brady brought home a kid; he was a freshman in high school that year. It was one of those 'Can he stay a day?' Well, then it'd end up two days. That one ended up five years. Well, in the meanwhile right after that one we had this other kid, he was a little older. ... 'Can Donny stay here for a night?' Two nights. We had him for five years. He didn't have nothing, no clothes or no nothing."

The Skramstads still scraped by for Les was disabled from diabetes in 1967 after a car fell on him at a mechanic's shop and damaged his pancreas—and they moved back to Libby. The things that held them together in tough times, Norita says, were simple: dinner and music. For a while Les and the boys supported the family with a small logging operation. They would come home hungry, Norita recalls, and she'd set out a big bowl of macaroni. "They were hungry so they'd fill up their plates, and by the time it got around to my daughter Sloan, she'd be like, 'There isn't going to be any left.' But there always was." Sharing precious food was only part of the equation. The table was the place where they talked. "Everything was discussed right at that kitchen table. Anything you wanted to know you heard, and maybe some things you didn't. Sloan, even about men things, she'd ask. And that's the way it was. They had no qualms about talking to us about anything. Even the girls: menstruation, boys, whatever. They talked with their dad just as well as they would me. They thought he was just as approachable as I was."

The second pillar of Skramstad family life was their music. It was there from the first, when Les and Norita were dating. "A lot of times, we'd just be sitting up there on the hill. Les was learning to play. We courted that way, with him strummin.' Forty-six years later I'm still kidding him about this. We've got pictures of me sitting there watching him learn how to play guitar." As their children grew, Les played bass and formed a band out of his progeny. The girls sang; Brady and Brent took up the guitar and drums. They even talked about having another child, this one a boy to be named Levi, to play fiddle. "Levi didn't have a chance," Les chuckles. Norita said five children were enough. Nevertheless the family band was a handy way of keeping track of them as they grew older. "We had the kids in the bars and I was a barmaid and Les was playing music. People would say, 'What are your kids doing in the bar?' I'd say, 'Well, where's your kids?' They were downtown, where? In the bar? Mine are right there. I know where they're at till 2 o'clock 'cause they're playing."

As Norita counts off her children's qualities—Laurel's endless affection, quiet Brent's thirst for perfection, Gayla's sentimentality,

Brady's charisma, and Sloan's love of the outdoors—Les chimes in occasionally, then abruptly leaves the room. Brent is sick with asbestosis; Norita and Laurel have been diagnosed. An initial exam showed Sloan had lung damage, but further tests have cleared her—so far. Les's rage is boundless. Some days he can talk about it, some days he is beyond words.

"That's the thing that bothers him the most is the fact that he brought it home," Norita says. "I told him, 'You know something that's going to hurt somebody, you'd want to tell them.' And here they didn't tell nobody. Plus the fact, the thing that bothers him the most is, he worked down near the ball fields, and during some of their experiments some of that stuff was sprayed out over towards the ball fields, in the shrubs. There's a lot of guilt. He'll just sit there and think about the kids. Of course they're all grown-up now, but how many of them played down there when I was doing that, and how many died?

"Now he'll sit sometimes and say, 'Did I do that to them?' Not knowingly, but still your mind will wonder. 'Did I do that to them?' The kids have been really good. They'll say, 'Hey, Dad, this has nothing to do with you.' And that does help, but it's still a fact. He gets to sitting there thinking, 'They were babies, just babies, when I brought it home.'"

Norita's instinct is to hold her own anger in check. "I try to balance it. I have a lot of anger like he does, but two angry people in a household won't work very good," she says. "We got some friends that are on both sides of it; they just fight over it. Even if they're on the same side, they both have it, they're at each other all the time." Plus she needs her energy to take care of Les, whose health is failing visibly month by month.

"It is kinda scary, mostly at night. You realize they're not breathing, you know," Norita says. "The first time I heard it I was afraid he wasn't going to breathe again because it just seemed like it was ten minutes. It's not, it's just seconds, but it seemed like it was forever before he gasped there and started breathing again. And he has trouble walking. He still tries to go outside and do things. It might take him all day but you can't just sit in the chair. ... If you look out he's probably sitting. He'll probably do something for five minutes and sit for half an hour, but he's still trying to do something other than just sit and doing nothing. That's good too. He has trouble walking; he walks sometimes like a drunken sailor. I try to nonchalantly watch him, make sure if we're out someplace … I don't know if you've ever noticed: he can't stand. He'll find something to lean against here. And I'll just nonchalantly walk close enough to him he can hang on to me or rest his arm or something. So I try to do it very discreetly, 'cause they don't like that.

"If he's by himself, sometimes he's talking to you and he'll walk clear over there and people think, 'Good Lord!' But he can't stand so he has to go over there where he can lean on something or sit. I know some people probably wonder, 'My Lord, why'd he go clear over here?' But he's got no balance."

The things Les used to do for fun—snowmobiling and carpentry work around the house—are long gone. He gave up hunting, he told lawyers at a deposition. After his accident in 1967, he'd found that life had become so precious, he couldn't take it from a deer. "I just quit that because it was too hard on me for one thing. And after being that close to losing my own life, I couldn't take another life."

While Earl Lovick went to his grave refusing to express remorse, Les atones for his children's illnesses, and for having sprayed asbestos near the ball fields where other people's children played, by fighting Grace for justice. "In a way, people say it keeps it fresh in his mind. Well yeah, it does. But still at the same time it gives him something positive to do. It's probably the best therapy," Norita says. "If he really gets upset, irate, he'll call Gayla, because we've known Gayla for so long. She's kinda like a sounding board. He can say whatever he wants to say, however he wants to say it, it will go no further. They have their chats, sometimes hour ones, but it works for him. I think sometimes that has been his biggest salvation is just being involved."

Winter is a hard season for people with asbestosis: the struggle of walking through the snow and balancing on ice, compounded by the shock of cold air on damaged lungs. So long as he is sitting,

Les looks as though he's not doing too badly yet this year, just before Christmas 2001. His daughter Gayla is visiting from North Carolina with her husband and little girl, McKenna, and Les's face glows as he talks of how happy his children make him. In a few days they'll all meet in Havre, a five-hour drive to the east, where three of the other kids live. As Les, Norita, and I talk, McKenna's father comes in the door and the four-year-old rushes to him, shouting "Daddy, Daddy, Daddy!" She clings to his left leg, an unconscious reenactment of the days when Les came home from work dusty with asbestos fibers. "She misses you, huh?" I say. "Yeah, she misses me," he replies wryly.

Brothers

Fred and Paul Miron are like mirrors reflecting two sides of the universe: night and day, good and evil, light and dark. One can hear it in their voices: Fred, the elder brother, talking of his life in the pleasant tone of a man who has enjoyed the beauty of the world; Paul, the younger, exiled forever from such lightheartedness by war, his voice echoing with the darkness of all he has seen—the worst of humanity that didn't end in Vietnam but persisted in a more subversive way in Libby. Still, they have always been close, tied to each other first by childhood and now by their mortality.

People say Fred has a photographic memory. Although his recall may not be perfect, Fred allows that his mind is pretty darn good. He demonstrates by describing the mill where he once worked for the W.R. Grace corporation practically down to the nuts and bolts. "I was a relief operator, so I knew every job that there was to do," he says. "I could replace any man at any time." He started off in the old wet mill, the first stop for the raw ore where it was processed by machines originally built for Minnesota's Mesabi Iron Range. "In that particular area, there was the three jigs, there was the 70-inch screen, and there were a set of spirals," he says. "They looked just like a big screw, like a spiral. There was water, and a certain amount of product was run down with the water. It worked like on a centrifugal basis, the lighter stuff going to the outside, the heavier stuff to the center, which was the waste."

From there the ore was put through a chemical bath. "It was a mixture of amine, which is an animal by-product; it's kinda like yellow lard. That was all dissolved in water, of course hot water. And then there was another component that went with it called black oil; it was like number 6 black crude oil. Ore would go through a device that would coat it with this oil and amine, which caused it to float. After it had been floated and the majority of the biotite and the green sand, and of course asbestos, were separated from it, it went through a bath of caustic soda to remove the amine and the oil. Then the water was wrung out of it in a machine that we had there. From there it went to the dry mill to some huge dry-ers that were big rotating horizontal dryers that were fired with oil. It would heat that ore up and get the rest of the moisture out, then it went upstairs and it was screened in the dry mill."

As he takes me through the process, he puts each man in his job, reciting obituaries for the dead: the guys who cleaned the tail-ings and mine-to-mill conveyor belts (one dead, one still alive); his foreman at the dry mill ("a miserable little slob, short, fat, and ugly and he wasn't in very good health"); his foreman at the load-ing facility ("I think he croaked. He was also in bad shape with the lungs, if I recall correctly. But I do have excellent recall. I'm known for that all my life"). There is a hint of humor in his voice, a Michigan accent gilded with the delight of remembering as he talks about the reasons that led him to Montana from the Mid-west. His father, an orphan, rode the rails during the Depression and never got his fill of the road. After his parents' marriage fell apart, Dad set out for Montana and Fred followed shortly after, at age seventeen.

"When I first went out there, Montana was for people like my-self who enjoy the out-of-doors. I've always been extremely inter-ested in wildlife, plant life, you know, the fauna, the flora, the ecology, everything," he says. "The Libby area was like going back in time seventy-five years. It was just great. I loved it." Though he has since moved back to Michigan, to the wild Upper Peninsula country, Fred says he misses the West. "I'd be there still had this not happened, I guarantee you."

As Fred followed his father, so Paul followed his brother out west, though the younger man's journey was less of a jaunt than a flight. "I had just come out of Vietnam and it was wintertime, so I didn't work that winter," Paul says. "I had always been close with my brother and he was up there, so when spring came I went out there. ... I spent two years in Asia and I wasn't feeling well. I was kinda run down. I thought working in that fresh air and doing some hard work would make me feel better."

Paul worked as a mucker in the wet mill, keeping the machines and screens clean. "I used hoses a lot and I used brushes sometimes. It was kind of a pretty wet environment," he says. "They had high-pressure sprays on the screens, you know. Later on I got to thinking asbestos was probably encapsulated in all that water that came off those high-pressure sprays. So whether it was wet or not, I believe you were breathing it, irregardless, you know."

Both brothers have been diagnosed with asbestosis. Fred suspected for nearly two decades that the dust had damaged his lungs, though he didn't get the word on paper until 2000. Paul, with no health insurance and no family aside from his brother, has moved into a home run by the Veterans Administration in Wisconsin. "Thank God I was really bashed around during the war," he says. "I've got Agent Orange and a bunch of other crap, so I won't have to worry about it."

Still, he is angry; the heat comes off his voice through the phone lines half a continent away. "They talk about Oklahoma City, the tragedy of that. There was men, women, and children killed here, innocent people. You don't hear nothing about that. And not one of them ever goes to prison. That's bull, you know? They're worried about Grace going bankrupt. My undying wish is that they go bankrupt or dissolve from the face of the earth."

THREE

The Family Business

SEVEN YEARS IN HIS GRAVE, industrialist J. Peter Grace still inspires great animosity for his life's work. When the eighty-one-year-old died in 1995 of lung cancer, he left as a legacy a multibillion-dollar chemical corporation and changes in the federal bureaucracy that reverberate in national politics to this day.

His story is no American dream, however. Peter Grace was born rich, the inheritor of his family's shipping company, one of the United States' first multinational corporations. The Grace company was an enterprise so well formed that by the time Peter came along, it practically lived and breathed of its own accord, demanding of its human officers the characteristics imbued by its founders: great attention to detail, familiarity with power, and boundless opportunism.

Though the company founders—brothers William Russell and Michael Grace—were Irish-born, W.R. Grace & Co. was an American venture. When at age nineteen William Grace first stepped onto the soil of Callao, Peru, in 1851, he began setting down roots; the family corporate tree grew inextricably with the political and commercial structures of South America, then branched north to the United States, exerting great influence there as well. According to one biographer, the brothers virtually built Peru and were a driving force in U.S. policy toward South America during the late 1800s, and in America's turn-of-the-century expansionism in general. "During the decade and a half on either side of the turn of the century, the United States projected itself dramatically beyond its borders and joined the ranks of the great powers in influencing world developments. Nowhere else was this vigorous American brand of imperialism more evident than in the Western

Hemisphere," writes professor Lawrence Clayton in his 1985 biography of William Grace. "Indeed, the prosaic trader, the flamboyant railroad builder, and the venture capitalist formed the cutting edge of American expansionism. William and Michael Grace were in the vanguard of that group."

Though the company started out as a trading house, Casa Grace moved naturally into shipping, exploiting the Peruvian trade in bird guano and nitrate of soda (an ingredient in gunpowder and later in artificial fertilizers). When the guano trade was tapped out, they turned to South America's other exports—rubber, sugar, and textiles—and in turn imported the lumber of the Pacific Northwest, the coal of Appalachia, and steel and other products of the industrial age. Eventually Grace's subsidiaries would fly airplanes; run a bank; make tacos, bubble wrap, and medical equipment.

The Grace lineage sounds biblical in recitation: Grace patriarch James, a modest landowner of 250 acres in Ireland, had three daughters and four sons: William Russell, Michael, Morgan, and lame John. William begat two sons, Joseph Peter and William Russell Jr. To Joseph was born a son, J. Peter, whom biographer Clayton says his father once described as being prone to "argue." The story of J. Peter Grace Jr., called Peter as his father before him was simply called Joe, evolves naturally from his predecessors. As the shipping industry declined, he cast about for a new focus and settled on chemicals. In the early 1950s, a decade or so before buying the Zonolite mines in Libby and South Carolina, Grace purchased the Davison Chemical Company and Dewey and Almy Chemical Company, and charted a new course for his grandfather's company that kept it at the pinnacle of the American financial and political worlds. As his grandfather and father before him ran with the likes of Grover Cleveland, Andrew Carnegie, and Teddy Roosevelt, Peter Grace counted the nation's powerful men among his friends, including President Ronald Reagan. Under his leadership, W.R. Grace & Co. ranked in the top 100 of the Fortune 500 from the list's inception in 1955 until nearly the end of the century when, in anticipation of an avalanche of asbestos-related lawsuits, Grace isolated its construction products division and declared it bankrupt.

Though the company is not a newcomer to scandal (in a pre-
cursor to the defense contractor scandals of the 1980s, when the
military paid $640 for a toilet seat and $349 for a hammer, William
Grace was upbraided in 1884 for charging the navy between 25
and 300 percent above market rates for "supplies of coal, wood,
flour and other staples," according to Clayton's biography), it's
Peter's name that has become synonymous with the moral failures
of Grace. First, there was his role as head of Ronald Reagan's con-
troversial Grace Commission. In this position, depending on one's
perspective, his mission was either to make the federal bureaucracy
more efficient or to slash those mechanisms designed to check the
inclinations of corporate America to excess and abuse. Then there
were his associations. Grace belonged to groups like the anticom-
munist Knights of Malta and the right-wing AmeriCares, dedicated to promoting procapitalist policy in South America. He
employed and advocated for a Nazi war criminal, a personal friendship expressed on an organizational level during World War II,
when several Grace managers in South America allied their sym-
pathies with Germany.

These relations earned Grace many antagonists, but probably
none are so well researched as a man named Dr. David Egilman.

"Lawyers get paid $500 an hour to make sure I'm an asshole, so
I really get vetted," he tells me when we first meet. "You can assume anything I tell you, I've got some basis for it." Egilman is a
professor at Brown University, a medical doctor, and to a west-
erner's eyes, the caricature of an East Coast liberal. When I walk
into the chaos that is Never Again Consulting's new office space
in the pretty little town of Attleboro, Massachusetts, it takes me a
while to figure out Egilman is not putting on a show just for me.
The man I take to be my host is heavyset and bearded, dressed in
a bright red polyester dashiki and maroon jogging pants with rac-
ing stripes. Later he informs me this is the outfit he wore when
W.R. Grace lawyers insisted on deposing him during an asbestos
lawsuit—for that occasion, he says, he added a pair of bright
yellow Tweety Bird slippers, a yarmulke, and a prayer shawl. When
I walk in, he is shouting over the speakerphone at a plaintiffs'

lawyer he's been working with on a tobacco lawsuit. He motions me to sit down. They are swearing at one another, apparently in negotiations over basketball tickets, but the conversation includes insults to each other's intellect and parentage. He hangs up abruptly and turns his attention to me. "Now what can I do for you?" he asks sharply. I repeat an e-mail message I sent him explaining that I want to know more about the Grace corporation and browse through his voluminous files on the company.

Gayla Benefield first told me of Egilman's existence. "I bought my computer and learned how to operate a computer because David Egilman was out there," she says. For a while, Egilman's Grace files were online, but access was iffy. Some days he'd make them available, some days not. When I first wrote him asking to look at them, he shot back a reply: "Who are you and what do you want with them?" Gayla tells me that if Egilman decides I'm okay, then I'm in. If he takes a dislike to me, too bad. By some stroke of luck, he lets me download some depositions but there is just too much for my computer to handle over the phone lines. I plan a visit in the middle of January 2002 and after threatening to cancel the interview at the last minute, Egilman decides he will give me an afternoon.

"Sophie!" he bellows, and a pretty young woman appears in the doorway. "Sit down if you've got a chance, so you can learn something. This is Sophie." He introduces us. He employs kids just out of high school, pays them well ("more than they'd make flipping burgers," he says defensively, when I joke about cheap labor), and in exchange for their research and technical skills, feels obliged to fill in whatever gaps were left in their high school education. I turn on the tape recorder and get ready for the lecture. What follows is a sort of disjointed rambling that takes us from South America during World War II to the halls of Congress and on to Libby.

"I'll tell you what I know and what I don't know. ... There's a report from the Bolivian military attaché that says [Grace] was the worst company with respect to Nazi cooperation. The Nazis were using Grace properties in Guatemala, and a lot of the Nazi propaganda that came into the United States came on Grace ships.

"So these are history lessons you should have learned in high school. So I have a lot of those state department documents, some of which were declassified only in the last five or six years. There's a whole set of other Nazi documents that were declassified within the last two years that are at the University of Maryland in Columbia, Maryland, that I haven't had a chance to look through.

"And some of these documents about their complicity with the Nazis, not only do they occur after the United States entered the war, *entered the war*—so a lot of the ones we have weren't declassified earlier because we were trying to protect Grace, understand? These would have hurt him when he was head of the Grace Commission. He was a big friend of Reagan, shit like that. So we've got a lot of documents from the Reagan papers too."

In fact, Egilman does have all these documents. The pattern they show is not so much active collaboration with Germany, but a certain tolerance for South American Nazis—a businessman's willingness to play both sides.

First there are two U.S. State Department memos written prior to America's entrance into World War II that finger Panagra—an airline half-owned by Grace—as the method of transport for Axis propaganda between Peru and the United States. After the U.S. entered the war, political and intelligence sources reported a number of connections between Grace personnel and suspected German Nazis, including the information that the Grace Line ship *Santa Lucia* was employing people with "Axis leanings." Similarly, a May 16, 1942, FBI report written by the ever-suspicious J. Edgar Hoover asserts that two Grace coffee farms in Guatemala were being managed by Germans.

As the war progressed, three men in Grace's employ aroused further suspicion on the part of the U.S. First there's the pilot Floyd E. Nelson. The FBI tailed him in 1942 when they suspected the man of espionage. "A close watch was kept on Panagra Pilot Nelson during the periods of his stays in Lima from April 30 to June 5, 1942. During this period he made about 150 contacts which might not be considered absolutely innocent, the majority of which are definitely suspicious, if not damning." This report, sent to the State Department by FBI director Hoover, includes an accounting of Nelson's rather active social life. Practically no one Nelson met with was beyond suspicion of Axis leanings in Hoover's analysis; however, the list reads like a who's who of the German community in Peruvian business and political circles.

In Bolivia, Grace's penchant for hiring family got them in trouble. Colonel Melitón Brito was the commercial manager for Panagra's Bolivia operations, a post he seemed to hold mainly because his father-in-law worked as Grace's lawyer. In 1942, Brito earned the enmity of the U.S. Embassy. "At the time we were trying to get undesirable Nazis deported for repatriation," reported embassy employee Allen Dawson to the U.S. Ambassador. "[T]he Government had sent a telegram to Col. Brito, the Prefect of Cochabamba asking him to detain and send up to La Paz several dangerous persons including one Hans Kempski. ... Brito had sent a telegram back to the effect that Kempski and the others were excellent persons who were a credit to Bolivia and not in any way engaged in dangerous activities." According to one of Dawson's agents, "Kempski is an exceptionally aggressive person with a type of personality that leaves little room for expansion beyond himself and his Nazi interests. His entire philosophy follows the basic tenet of the Nazis 'to live but let nothing else live.' His conversations are all from the totalitarian point of view. There is little question but that he is a dangerous Nazi."

Earning Grace additional hostility were the actions of the company's general manager in Bolivia. For reasons unexplained, people seemed to hate Julio Guzmán Tellez. U.S. military attaché Clarence Barnett wrote on January 26, 1942, that Tellez

> is an opportunist of the worst type. He is a Bolivian Citizen, Manager of an American firm who has no loyalty to either government ... there have been many shady deals attributed to Dr. Guzmán Tellez and it is certain that some of them are true, however, Grace officials say that "he is a Bolivian and a politician and knows how to handle the Bolivians and in addition makes money for us." This is of course typical of W.R. Grace & Company throughout South America. If there is a worst [sic]

company in the United States than W.R. Grace & Company it
would be interesting to hear of it. No actual Pro-Nazism can be
proven against Dr. Guzmán Tellez, but neither can any Pro-
American actions be proven in his favor.

Egilman came by all these papers by accident, he says. The doctor has made a sideline testifying on behalf of plaintiffs' lawyers in
so-called toxic torts cases, taking on asbestos and tobacco companies among others. In one of these cases, Grace lawyers insisted
and the judge agreed that Egilman should produce evidence supporting every one of his statements against the asbestos companies.
The resulting document he labeled "Kevorkia," because he considered it suicidal for Grace to make such a request.

"I didn't know much about them until these depositions," he
says. "They were trying to harass me; they did ten days of deposition, videotaped me. And they asked me when I went to temple,
and how often I wore a yarmulke. Those kind of harassing questions about my personal life, I don't think I should answer those
questions.

"Someone like me understands that if you harass me success-
fully, then that's going to tell all these other companies I'm doing
research on to harass me. ... [Grace] was always sending me things
and asking for stuff, and every time they asked a question I'd go
find out the answer. That's bad for them because most of the
answers are bad for them. Okay, you see all these answers? I didn't
know any of this shit until they started asking me questions, right?"

In the process of all this research, Egilman came across a 1987
deposition taken in an Alaska district court of a Grace employee
named Arnold Rosenberg. A statement on page 75 caught his
attention. The attorney asked Rosenberg to identify the author of
a 1972 memo, a Grace consultant. "The memorandum also refers
to Dr. Ambrose," the lawyer stated. "Who was Dr. Ambrose?"

"That is a real interesting question," Rosenberg replied. "Otto
Ambrose was part of Hitler's group, and I think he was called the
'Devil's Chemist.' ... And, since he had been part of the group
that had put together the German chemical industry, Peter Grace

hired him as a consultant to Grace Chemicals when Grace got into chemicals. As a matter of fact, I think he's the one who suggested to Peter Grace that 'If you want to spend some money, get into the chemical business.'"

Egilman finds this phrasing hilarious. "The answer was, he was one of Hitler's boys, like he played for Harvard? Okay? You know, some people they played for Yale, some people they played for Tufts, they got a football team? U Mass, University of Montana, and then some people played for Hitler." But the Nazi connection struck an obvious chord with Egilman. His father survived Germany's concentration camps, though Felix Egilman lost his first wife and set of children to the Nazis. In a November 2001 interview with *Rhode Island Monthly* magazine, Egilman recalls the darkness of his childhood. "My father was not a very nice person. … He had not had a very good life. He worked, and after work he peddled shoes. We didn't have much to talk about."

German chemist Otto Ambrose first made the acquaintance of American scientists when the Allied forces sent a team of agents to the small town of Gendorf, Bavaria, near the Auschwitz concentration camp in May 1945. According to Linda Hunt, a former CNN reporter and author of the book *Secret Agenda*, about the U.S. government's Project Paperclip efforts to bring German scientists to America after the war, "The team's mission was to capture and interrogate Hitler's scientists, locate and microfilm documents, and confiscate all useful equipment found in laboratories and factories."

This particular Allied team had targeted an I.G. Farben chemical plant on the outskirts of town and smashed through the gates with a Sherman tank, Hunt writes. "The spoils … discovered at Gendorf included some of the greatest scientific minds in Hitler's chemical warfare industry. One was Walter Reppe, an I.G. Farben director and pharmaceutical research expert. Even more impressive was Otto Ambrose, a well-known chemist and Farben director who had come to Gendorf to construct a rubber plant nearby." Ambrose, as it turned out, was later described in a U.S. intelligence document as "the key man in German Chemical Warfare production."

But at first, no one had any idea as to Ambrose's importance. Nuremberg prosecutor Josiah DuBois, who wrote a book on Farben's scientists called *The Devil's Chemists*, reported that Ambrose came off initially as a folksy, friendly guy. "He passed soap out to the soldiers personally—it was good to have somebody dropping gifts in their hands for a change. The brass felt the same way when he issued cleaning agents and paints for the vehicles. They were not scientists but any scientist worth his salt could talk about technical things simply and with a smile. This fellow Ambrose could tell you how to make a hundred wonderful products from one chemical element, ethylene oxide." And, DuBois added, "he knew more about rubber than anything else."

In fact, Ambrose had led a team that discovered a new way to make synthetic rubber, called Buna, earning Hitler's praise and a prize of one million deutsche marks. In the courtroom, DuBois learned the story behind the Buna plant at Gendorf. "To the inmates of Camp I, the word 'Buna' ... was more frightful than 'Auschwitz'— the Farben site more terrifying than any place except a large wooden area three kilometers east of Camp I." Survivors described the scene for Nuremberg justices: "The prisoners ... who were given easier jobs remembered better and longer than most," DuBois wrote. "The inmates were forced to carry one-hundred C-weight bags of cement. 'It took four men to lift one bag and put it on the back of one man. When the inmates couldn't go along quick enough to satisfy the Farben *Meister*, the *Meister* beat them with sticks and iron bars and punched them with his fists and kicked them. I have often seen them beaten to death with iron bars.'"

Ambrose was the director of this factory, which used free men as well as prisoners in its labor force. He was by all accounts an accomplished chemist, credited with being part of the team who discovered the nerve gases Sarin and Tabun. His Farben plant also manufactured Zyklon-B, which was used in the gas chambers. U.S. intelligence documents report that Ambrose was accused of having tested the efficiency of his gases on Auschwitz inmates. In 1948 he was convicted of slavery and mass murder, for which he served three years in prison. When he was released in 1951, he went to work for Peter Grace under the protection of a program called Project National Interest, which according to reporter Linda Hunt's research, matched up Nazis, among others, with jobs at U.S. corporations and universities.

The relationship with Otto Ambrose was an important one to Peter Grace, testified Bradley Dewey Jr., son of the founder of Dewey and Almy, in 1996. "Otto Ambrose was a consultant to Grace. And particularly to Peter. And Peter would often ask Dr. Ambrose for his judgment. It was in my interest to have Dr. Ambrose aboard when I as President of the Cryovac Division wanted something that perhaps Peter wanted some other input on."

"It was in your interest to get Dr. Ambrose to agree with your position?" the lawyer asked.

"I wanted him on my side. And we had a mutual friendship. He helped quite a lot. He brought some German technology into focus for me which we were able to buy which was important at one stage of our development. Technology having to do with making plastic films."

"Was it your impression that Mr. Grace valued Dr. Ambrose's views on matters?" the lawyer asked.

"Very much," Dewey replied. Dewey told the lawyers that he met with Ambrose in Germany once or twice a year, and that Ambrose couldn't come to the United States.

The lawyer asked why.

"He was a very proud man. He had been convicted at the Nuremberg trials. Spent time in jail. The Jewish lobby was out to get him. He wasn't going to be exposed to that. ... I have been told that he couldn't get a visa."

Grace did try to get a visa for his new consultant. According to the diary of the U.S. ambassador to Germany, David Kirkpatrick Bruce, Grace came by for lunch on July 22, 1958, to discuss the matter. "[Grace] is the active head of the far-flung Grace enterprises," Bruce wrote. "The reason for his visit was to try to obtain assistance for the grant of a visa to Dr. Otto Ambrose, a distinguished German scientist once in prison as a Director of IGF for the use of slave labor during the war. I told him I would check with the consulate General at Stuttgart on the status of the case." Grace followed up with a letter to the U.S. Consul in Stuttgart, Germany, asking that the doctor be given a visa to attend a technical meeting in the United States. Press reports quote the letter as stating, "During the seven years we have known Dr. Ambrose and have had the opportunity of working with him, we have developed a very deep admiration not only for his ability, but more important for his character in terms of truthfulness and integrity."

Grace lawyers have in recent years declared that "Grace has no information that [Ambrose] had any dealings with Grace (or any business connected to Grace) concerning asbestos or fireproofing, with the possible exception that in 1972 he may or may not have met with Dr. Preston Veltman, then a Grace employee, to discuss Monokote." In fact, internal company papers document that Grace sent Ambrose regular reports in the early 1970s that dealt in part with the asbestos-laden Monokote insulation, and that were to be distributed on a "real need to know" basis. Also, Grace apparently consulted with Ambrose prior to its purchase of Zonolite on the question of what to do with Libby's "tramp" asbestos: "Ideally we should seek to use present Zonolite discard streams for filling voids in the exfoliated structure. The possibility of utilizing the short-fibered asbestos for this purpose should be considered. ... Zonolite may be a preferred material around which to develop an inorganic foam. Ambrose and others believe that a reasonably priced product of this kind would have real sales potential."

All this information became news when Reagan appointed Peter Grace to head up the Grace Commission. Egilman credits a congressman, a Democrat from California named Tom Lantos, with making Grace and Ambrose's friendship a public scandal. "Tom Lantos couldn't take a joke. You know who Tom Lantos is? He was a congressman, and the reason he couldn't take a joke is because he was in a concentration camp. See? So he didn't think it was funny that Grace was using a convicted Nazi war criminal as a consultant, particularly because that particular Nazi war criminal ran the Auschwitz death camp. Okay? [Where] probably some of his relatives, maybe he was even at. So he didn't think that was funny. Had no sense of humor whatsoever. Just a convicted mass murderer and slaver.

"Or as the Grace lawyer said to me, 'Dr. Egilman, he served his time. Don't you think that he should be rehabilitated now and we should be able to use him?' To which I responded, 'Well, it doesn't matter very much what I think. The United States Congress has decided that convicted Nazi war criminals can never come to this country. So we kind of made that decision as a society.'

"Here's a funny Dewey story. I got to give you this quote, because this is one of my favorite quotes. You won't believe it unless I find it." He rummages around his computer files, looking for Dewey's deposition. On page 76, the lawyer asks Dewey if he knows what Ambrose had been convicted of.

"I believe it had to do with the part he played in reaching the decision to build a synthetic rubber plant near Auschwitz which would employ as labor persons headed to Auschwitz who were too healthy to go right to the gas chambers," Dewey replied.

Again Egilman starts laughing. "Don't you think that's funny?

"That was his job. That was Bradley Dewey's definition of Otto Ambrose's job. That was his job, because you wouldn't want to send someone who was too healthy to the gas chamber. Right? You'd want to work them until they were sick, wouldn't you? As an efficient person?"

Egilman is getting wound up, warming into a rant.

"You wouldn't want to send them with their gold teeth, you wouldn't want to send them with their hair, you wouldn't want to bury them with their skin. All that shit's usable, right? Window shades, shades on your lamps, lamp shades, you know, you ought to recycle that shit. Look at all the people into recycling. They were just ahead of their time. See? They were into recycling skin. We're into that now. They were just ahead of that. Ahead of his time, Otto Ambrose. So that's one of my favorite quotes. You know, because I never really conceived of that concept. Anytime somebody opens you up to a new idea, it's important.

"Don't you think that's funny?" Sophie and I squirm a bit. I nod, acknowledging the sarcasm, encouraging him to move on.

"Now she's here," he's says to Sophie, pointing at me, "because Grace killed a bunch of people up in Libby, Montana. These miners, they'd work all day, come home at night dusty with asbestos, *and their little kids would get to breathe it in too.* Don't you think that's funny?"

I am startled when the image of Les and Norita Skramstad's granddaughter McKenna hanging on her father's legs comes vividly to my mind. Suddenly I understand the attempt at false humor is a facade hiding the depth of his rage, and I taste the bitterness driving his rhetorical questions. No, it's not funny. It's not funny at all.

To be fair, W.R. Grace was not the only corporation to employ Ambrose. According to documents from former president Reagan's archives, he worked as well for Dow Chemical and the U.S. Department of Energy. And, as Linda Hunt reports in her book, in 1957 W.R. Grace was just one of sixty companies involved in Project National Interest: participants included the likes of Lockheed, Martin-Marietta, and CBS Laboratories.

In this context, one could argue, Grace was just another all-American company.

THE FIRST FOUR MONTHS OF 1963 were exciting ones for the Zonolite Corporation: By April, the Chicago men who had turned Ed Alley's small enterprise into an international business had negotiated the sale of the Libby operation, along with another vermiculite mine in Enoree, South Carolina, to the much larger W.R. Grace corporation in a stock-for-stock transaction (with four shares of Zonolite stock traded in for each share of Grace stock). But for Grace the process began much earlier than the sale date.

According to a 1962 document entitled "Acquisition of Zonolite Company," Libby's asbestos was actually a draw for the multinational company. "In Zonolite's Montana ore deposits, tremolite asbestos occurs in varying concentrations. There are rich veins containing up to 80 percent asbestos which are discarded as mine waste," the report begins. "The asbestos volume available is believed adequate to support a commercial recovery rate of 50,000 tons per year and pilot work is under way on a process for so doing." The report goes on to note that Zonolite had been buying commercial asbestos to mix in with its products rather than using the stuff on hand from the mine. The writers speculate that not only could Zonolite save money by using its own asbestos, but tremolite could have commercial potential on its own as well. "It is believed that the tremolite type asbestos can be substituted for enough of the 1961 estimated U.S.A. consumption of 490,000 tons of short fiber chrysotile asbestos to provide an attractive market (at $40 a ton) for the proposed Libby asbestos mill." The report predicts $300,000 in post-tax earnings for Libby's potential asbestos operations by the year 1966.

Libby was not Grace's first foray into the asbestos market, nor was it the corporation's first experience with asbestos-related diseases. When Peter Grace bought Dewey and Almy Chemical in 1953 and took on Bradley Dewey Sr. as a senior consultant, he gained the benefit of Dewey's extensive knowledge on the subject. At least as early as the 1930s, Dewey and Almy was experimenting with asbestos in its rubber and plastics products. Among its operations was the manufacture of synthetic rubber, Buna, the demand for which reached a fevered pitch during the war. (Buna, of course, was one of Otto Ambrose's specialties.) By the late 1930s, this line had led to a debate among Dewey, his insurance company, and a Boston Department of Labor official over whether all kinds of asbestos were equally toxic. Dewey, having studied the question, knew enough about asbestos-related diseases to be of the opinion that some fibers were worse than others. He explained himself in a 1938 letter:

> 1. As I understand it, Multibestos ran for years without much trouble. It then switched to Russian and Rhodesian crudes and suffered an enormous amount of trouble.
> 2. I have been through plants of competitors ... where conditions have been so bad that vision from one end of the shop to the other was actually impaired by asbestos dust in the air. In some of these, long streamers of asbestos fiber hung from every beam, sprinkler pipe and shaft hanger. Where these plants

reported no trouble, I could not help but be impressed by the fact
that they had seemed to have a long history back of them of having
used only Canadian fiber.

3. It seemed to me that in many of the cases where I had heard
that the plants had suffered trouble, they were the ones that had
used goodly quantities of foreign fibers.

4. I personally cannot study the disease record of the Walpole
plant and not believe that asbestosis is a very serious and sometimes fatal disease.

Thirty years later, Grace would pronounce the Libby asbestos
pilot project a failure: tremolite fibers proved weaker than the
commercial chrysotile asbestos, and freight was simply too expensive for Libby's asbestos to compete with soil conditioners like
diatomaceous earth. At that point, however, Grace could not have
been too dismayed. The mid-1960s were record years for the company, with sales and revenues exceeding $1 billion in 1965, in-
creasing another 17 percent in 1966, and again in the first half of
1967. And Libby certainly added to these numbers: in 1968 the
mine was supplying 67 percent—267,000 tons—of the "free
world's total vermiculite," according to an internal Grace review
of Libby's ore body. Most of it went to markets in the United States
and Canada. Though expensive to recover and ship, Libby's mine
was full of high-grade vermiculite, the report concluded, enough
to last at least another seventy-five or one hundred years.

While the accountants' ledgers failed to show that the true price
of those profits was eating away at the miners' lungs, by the late
1960s Grace executives were well aware of the problem. In fact,
between annual X-ray and lung function tests and a number of
studies commissioned by the corporation, Grace officials could
have predicted which men were going to die of asbestos-related
diseases long before many of these workers even realized they were
sick. To look at all those documents, medical tests, and internal
discussions is to realize that the Grace corporation's actions in
Libby amounted to one big medical experiment, with the townspeople serving as unwitting laboratory rats.

Some Kind of Friend

It's a good thing Earl Lovick was already dead and buried when Louise McNair found out he had stolen her late husband's lungs. "He was supposed to have been a real good friend of ours. Had my husband taking him fishing at a private lake we took care of part of the time," she says, fuming. "That's the kind of horse's ass he was."

Louise met her future husband, Michael McNair, at a tender age even for those days. The daughter of homesteaders, she grew up in Rexburg, Montana, a town that now lies under the water backed up by the Libby dam. Michael was a friend of her brother-in-law's. "I was only about fourteen but he didn't know that. He thought I was older because my sister, who was married to my brother-in-law, was six years older than I, and that's what he thought I was." Three years later they eloped, eluding friends who tried to stop them in Libby, by sneaking off to Kalispell and lying about Louise's age.

Michael McNair, described by his friends as one of the most competent woodsmen they'd ever met, went to work for Zonolite in 1942 when his oldest daughter was six months old. Before that, he had worked summers for the Forest Service, then as a trapper in the winter. "He more than doubled his money [as a trapper] than when he was alternate ranger in the summertime for the Forest Service, which I wish he would have stayed at," Louise says. Instead he strung the first telephone line up to the mine site, then went to work in Grace's mechanics shop. He moved his family into one of the five cabins the company kept for employees on Rainy Creek Road, and his next three children were born there. "We lived in Zonolite Canyon for three years, when they had houses up there," Louise recalls. "The whole yard was Zonolite. We didn't have a lawn."

Now all four of the McNair children are sick with what Louise calls "the Zonolite." She has asbestosis as well and steadfastly refuses to accept any visitors because of it. "I'm not too well and I have a real hard time walking or sitting or anything because of this," she explains, insisting on a phone interview.

When Michael died in 1983, Louise says, she wanted to know what killed him, so she ordered an autopsy to be performed in Kalispell. "Lovick found out about it, so he grabbed the lung and headed back east," she says. A Grace memorandum dated October 18, 1983, describes the company's findings: "Uncoated total fiber content of the lung was 49.7 million fibers per gram of dry tissue. 87% of this fiber was tremolite or tremolite containing some iron which he calls tremolite actinolite," wrote Grace safety director Harry Eschenbach, quoting the doctor, Patrick Sebastien, who dissected the lung. "[Sebastien] indicates that an average person would have far less than one million fibers per gram of dry tissue. ... Patrick pointed out that the uncoated fiber size distribution in McNair's lung was remarkably similar to that which he found in analyzing air samples from Libby."

FOUR
Mountain of Grace

THE HOTEL ROOM is stuffy with recycled air from the heater, a shield against the winter weather outside. It's my first introduction to Les Skramstad, a slight man who this evening just before Christmas 1999 wears a gray complexion that matches the season and is clearly uncomfortable in the closed space. Yet he; his wife, Norita; and their friend Gayla Benefield have insisted on this meeting late tonight. They sit facing me like a panel of judges, though I'm the one asking questions. The tape recorder chews through cassette after cassette. I am coming down with a cold, and the evening weighs heavy on me. But Gayla and the Skramstads have come down with something much worse, a modern plague that will rob them and at least three of their collective children of a full life. They know now, maybe decades ahead of time, how their death certificates will read: pulmonary fibrosis, lung cancer, or mesothelioma. The diseases of asbestos.

We get to know each other slowly. I ask about work and their kids. But this is no small talk. Les worked for two and a half years for the company mining on Vermiculite Mountain, first putting in his time sweeping the dusty dry mill. Later, Les transferred into town where he crawled around on his hands and knees, separating impurities from the piles of pure asbestos fibers his bosses wanted to experiment with. That was forty years ago, and in the meantime he supported his family working as an auto mechanic, playing electric bass on the weekends for a country band called the Sundowners. For the sake of those few paychecks early in his married life, he's dying now, without insurance, unable to work. But the worst of it is, so are his wife and two of his five children. He can barely speak for the weight of his guilt, so Gayla chimes in.

"What person doesn't set out to protect his family? I mean, this man here would give his life for his family."

The snow has turned to rain outside, and we sit listening to its drumming on the pavement. "It's a heavy cross to bear," Les finally says.

After the three leave, I sit typing my notes late into the night. They've lain out a map for me, an outline of a mystery that seems to touch the very central questions of human existence: Why did W.R. Grace let its workers be poisoned? Who are these people who can make such decisions? Is there redemption in death for guilt such as Grace's? For the anger Les Skramstad carries? The answers must lie where it all began, on Grace's mountain.

Vermiculite Mountain rises to a modest 4,200 feet, a smallish, unremarkable hill compared with the spectacular ice and rocks of nearby Glacier National Park. Many of the peaks and valleys in the surrounding Kootenai National Forest have been logged, with clear-cuts lining the road for most of the 90 miles east to Kalispell, the region's largest town. It was a fate escaped by Vermiculite Mountain while its owners were busy extracting ore. Now that the cut has declined on public lands and the mine has closed, loggers have begun to work this hill as well.

EPA toxicologist Chris Weis agrees to be my guide to the mountain the morning after my meeting with Gayla, Les, and Norita, though he is practically a tourist himself. Weis is part of the agency's emergency response team sent from Denver, which swooped down on Libby like a SWAT team within a week of the dire reports in a Seattle newspaper breaking the story that 200 people of this town had been killed, and possibly thousands more made sick, while no one from any level of government paid any attention.

Weis picks a chunk of ore out of the trunk of his rental car to show me. "Looks like coyote scat, doesn't it?" And it does—remarkably so. Weis has parked halfway up the dirt road to the mine and is pointing out landmarks. Across the ravine is the old tailings pile, where miners dumped waste rock. Practically a mountain in itself, the terraced pile supports scraggly clumps of grass and not much else. The hill slopes down to Rainy Creek, where a half-dozen ducks float on one of two ponds created by a mud dam, a system engineered to keep mine waste out of the nearby Kootenai River. The lowland is lush with cattails and willows, and an osprey nest suggests the presence of trout. "This is actually a very healthy wetland," Weis says. "I wish all mine closures were as good-looking as this one."

But looks are deceiving. By Weis's calculations, the amount of tremolite asbestos in that tailings pile ranges from 30 to 40 percent. These ponds are most certainly contaminated, he allows. Asbestos washed—still washes during flood season—downstream into the river and beyond.

"We can't go all the way up—it's private land," he says, pointing to the top of the hill where the actual mine was. "But on a clear day, you can stand on top and see town."

Pink flags line the dirt road every 1,000 feet or so down to the river marking the EPA's sampling sites. Extra flags dot the "amphitheater," a clearing by the side of the road where trucks hauling ore down to the river could turn off to let one another pass, used until now by high school kids for weekend keg parties. Grace stored vermiculite, graded by size, in a series of bins and silos on the west side of the river. When the time came to load the ore for shipping by rail to expansion plants across the country, an operator would pull a switch, dumping a mess of it onto an underground conveyor belt that emerged from the riverbank and crossed the water to the old Burlington Northern railroad tracks on the east side. On a bench just above the tracks, a developer has plans to build a subdivision. Another set of flags marks the grounds where the old storage and loading facility sat, currently occupied by a family-owned nursery. The business, which sold houseplants to the EPA to help brighten up the agency's spartan office, would be forced to shut down several months later, after the officials declared the grounds to be highly contaminated. On into town, the agency has flagged baseball fields that adjoin more processing facilities.

In the early months of 2000 the EPA will find that all the mining facilities are contaminated with asbestos. Preliminary results show tremolite in the dust along Rainy Creek Road, in the tunnels at the loading facility, the old expansion plant downtown near the Little League baseball fields.

But that's not all.

Vermiculite mining was a dusty business, and for the nearly 70-year life span of the mine the workers went home filthy each night. Employees were told the asbestos-laden dirt was "nuisance dust," and their wives breathed it in as they scrubbed clothing and curtains and floors. Their children inhaled it as they played on the carpet. Their neighbors got a dose when they put vermiculite in their gardens and insulation from the mine into their attics. Vacuuming simply tossed the tremolite fibers into the air, where they settled at a rate of one foot per hour.

When news of dead and dying townspeople with no connection to the mine finally hit the media in 1999, Grace CEO and chairman Paul Norris responded with a press release saying, "We were surprised to learn of the allegations since no one had raised them with us previously." His point man, Alan Stringer, seconded and clarified Norris's statement. "Sure, I knew that there were issues with past workers and workers' families. This is a small town and for people to deny that they didn't know that is a little shortsighted," he told me. "I knew it, but I didn't believe that there was a problem to the town in general from past or current operations."

But Grace's dust ignored artificial boundaries, obeyed no property lines, and corporate managers knew this. When the winds blew right, the nearly constant dust cloud from the dry mill drifted into town. In a 1965 memo, one Grace supervisor wrote, "Butch thinks you could get a 5 count in downtown Libby on many dry days." Former Grace manager Earl Lovick interpreted this for lawyers during a 1997 deposition: Butch was Libby manager Raymond "Butch" Bleich, and a "5 count" translated to 5 million particles of dust per cubic foot. One of Grace's own engineers estimated the asbestos content of the dry mill dust at 12 to 23 percent, dust that was exhaled outside the mill by huge fans, then left to the whims of the prevailing winds. Added up, this means Libby's citizens working or shopping downtown were breathing air that contained between 600,000 and more than 1 million particles of asbestos fibers per cubic foot of air.

In 1967, Grace measured the dust coming out of one stack and found that it spewed out about 12 tons of airborne particulate matter a day. While state law allowed less than 1 ton of such discharge per day, Lovick said he could recall no effort on the part of Montana officials to enforce the law.

Likewise, court documents reveal that Grace and its Libby employees did nothing to discourage a long-established practice whereby Libby folks went down to the Grace expanding plant, or out to the loading facility, and hauled pickup truck loads of waste vermiculite—ore that wasn't quite up to standards for commercial use—and took it home to put in between their walls as insulation and in their gardens to break up the hard clay soil. This went on with Grace's tacit approval and continued until the mine closed in 1990.

The EPA tested fifty-two homes in the first months of 2000, taking soil and insulation samples and pumping air through a high-tech vacuum system. The results: more than half of these, twenty-seven homes, had asbestos in the air or dirt, with four of these registering tremolite at dangerous levels. Test results were still pending for Libby's schools, with more aggressive sampling scheduled for the summer months. Eventually, EPA technicians would find still more asbestos under the high school and middle school running tracks, in the grade school skating rink, and hear rumors of it—gossip that would thankfully turn out to be false— lying in the corner of a preschool playground. But by the summer of 2000, the conclusions were clear: ten years after the mine closed, Libby residents were still being poisoned by asbestos from Zonolite Mountain. Members of at least two generations of Libby residents, perhaps more, could expect to die from the mine's airborne dust.

MAPS ARE A PART OF LIFE IN rural Montana. With property lines patterned like a checkerboard, our maps tell us where we can hunt and hike. They delineate our neighbor's ranch from land

given to the railroads in 1864, delivered to subsidiary logging operations during the late 1980s, and reserved by the state and various
federal agencies for the public. Nearly 8.3 million acres of Montana
are owned by the public, though that fact has not been the cause
for rebellion that has erupted in other Rocky Mountain states
mainly because public land means hunting and access to fishing
holes, and opportunities for mushrooming and berry picking. As
much as some Montanans may gripe about restrictions on logging
or quarter granted to endangered species, we love and use our land;
we all have a stash of maps, and the contours of the country are as
clear in our minds as the lines of topography on paper.

So it is to maps that officials have turned to sort out the mess in
Libby. Soon after reports of the dead and dying hit the news, the
EPA emergency response team set up shop in a small storefront on
the town's main street, Mineral Avenue. The walls of the temporary office are covered; members of the crew encourage longtime
residents to drop by and pinpoint the landmarks of their memories. Here were the piles of vermiculite, here we separated the ore
into grades, this was the route we hauled it to town, where bags of
Zonolite were loaded onto the old Burlington Northern line and
shipped all over the country.

To say that the man in charge of these maps is out of place in
Libby is an understatement. Paul Peronard is unmistakably a city
boy with tattoos, pierced ears, and shaven head. But he has a
steadiness about him, a confident, straightforward manner that
conveys both credibility and openness. These characteristics have
served him well with the media and with the town's asbestos victims. The others—the local car salesmen, realtors, and retailers
who make up the Chamber of Commerce crowd—have taken to
calling him Paul Paranoid, and find their opinions—mainly that
everyone should just shut up about the problem before it hurts
Libby's economy—are eclipsed by the young man's charisma.

Peronard has got a formidable task: seeking out and cleaning up
as much of Libby's asbestos as possible. Just locating the so-called
hot-spots is a chore, when many people fear the consequences of
inviting the feds into their homes and lives. Plus so many of the

players in this decades-old drama are dead: the miners, of course, but also the doctors, the corporate officials, those paid to carry out company policy. It was a point finally driven home for me when I first called Grace spokesperson Alan Stringer on the telephone while working on a story about Libby for *Mother Jones* magazine. Stringer had recently moved back to Libby, where he raised his family working as a foreman from 1981 through the mine's closure in 1990. Now he acts as Grace's point man on the controversy. He can speak to those years he spent at the mine, he tells me, but refuses to answer questions about what happened in the early days. I ask him to give me a name or two, someone who could give an accounting for his employer during the 1960s and 1970s. His response, and the hysterical edge to his voice, are shocking: "You can't talk to them, they're all dead!" In fact, at least three Grace officials from the Libby days are still alive: a safety director/toxicologist named Harry Eschenbach, former mine manager Bill McCaig, and researcher Julie Yang. Efforts to reach Eschenbach at his home in Topsfield, Massachusetts, were unsuccessful. McCaig did not return phone calls or respond to letters sent to him in North Carolina. Stringer refused to go on the record with me after our initial conversation, and current Grace officials, including CEO Paul Norris, declined to grant any interviews at all. Only Yang was willing to talk about her limited experiences looking at Libby's air and ore samples under the microscope.

With time we've lost nearly all but the historical record, a paper trail of culpability where once living, breathing humans made choices for reasons we may never understand, and the consequences of which will reverberate here for generations.

THE CLUES TO LIBBY'S future filtered out slowly in the early years. The first indication of any problem at Zonolite actually surfaced in the early 1940s, when an inspector from the state warned Zonolite officials repeatedly that they needed to install dust control equipment. The inspector recommended that the miners be provided with respirators, though he stated that since the dust contained little or no silica, it was "classified as a nuisance dust."

That phrase—"nuisance dust"—was a crutch that Grace officials would lean on through the late 1970s to deflect questions about the dust, long after they knew it was full of asbestos.

Then there is no news for a dozen years, and there might never have been more except for the steadfast efforts of one man, a state health inspector named Ben Wake.

Before Peronard and his team rode into Libby in their white SUVs, before the headlines and court cases, even before the first dead miner, Wake filed his first report outlining the asbestos problem at the mine. It was 1956, seven years before Zonolite would sell out to the Grace corporation. State officials did something that would establish a pattern for the next three decades: they marked the report "Confidential"; Zonolite managers said nothing about the substance of its contents to their employees.

Wake, now retired and living in Salt Lake City, did not respond to a request for an interview. He likewise was not interested in helping out the asbestos victims' lawyers when they came calling. But his reports speak for themselves. All through the 1960s, he pursued Grace doggedly, using his inspection reports to map out a scenario of death and deceit that would last through time and, at the turn of the century, finally lead investigators to W.R. Grace's doorstep.

Ben Wake must have been a thorough man in his younger days. He covered considerable ground in that first report on Zonolite's operations. Floor by floor, he analyzed the dust in the dry mill, summarized and footnoted a study that compared the pathological changes in miners' lungs due to asbestos fibers with those arising from silica exposure. He explained how federal health recommendations are arrived at, how to calculate a man's exposure over an entire workday: "Weighted average exposures more nearly represent a workers actual exposure over an eight-hour day than does a single sample result representing an exposure for a short portion of an hour a day," he told a trio of plant managers, Butch Bleich, Earl Lovick, and Walter Baker. He concluded, "the asbestos dust in the air is of considerable toxicity, and is a factor in the consideration of reducing dustiness in the plant." Wake found dust concentrations in the dry mill as high as 83 million particles per cubic foot (mppcf), and estimated that, based on the company's records, between 8 and 21 percent of that dust was composed of asbestos fibers. This means the asbestos levels reached as high as 17 mppcf. The so-called maximum allowable concentration for asbestos, he told the managers, was 5 mppcf. Zonolite's men were breathing at least three times that amount. (In those days, analytical techniques were such that scientists couldn't count the number of asbestos fibers in air samples, but instead extrapolated from bulk ore samples the percentage of asbestos in the air, expressed as part of the total dust count.)

In fact, Wake misunderstood the industry standards. The U.S. Public Health Service (relying on a 1938 asbestos report by former U.S. surgeon general Waldemar Dreessen) appears to have intended the 5-million-particle standard to apply to the total dust count—in which case Libby's miners were breathing more than thirteen times the industry's "safe" level.

Wake's first report includes two and a half pages' worth of recommendations. Because the paper was marked "Confidential," the information went no further.

More reports followed further inspections. Wake had been relying in his analysis on company assurances that the quantity of asbestos in Libby's ore ranged from 10 to 20 percent. But in 1962 he received a shock. Wake had sent samples to the federal Public Health Service for testing with an explanation: "We are enclosing with the dust sample two samples of raw material which may aid you in the analysis. The smaller piece of granular nature with little of the white material mixed in is what would be called at the plant a good project material of vermiculite and would be a high-grade ore. The white material is, we understand, a type of asbestos which is a contaminant in the product and runs about ten percent at the most in the raw feed of the plant. ... The plant expects, in the near future, to begin milling the lower grade ore which would, of course, increase the air-borne dust concentrations substantially."

One month later, the Public Health Service wrote Wake, informing him that the asbestos content of that "high-grade ore" was

40 percent—two to four times what Zonolite had told him. Wake passed this information along to Zonolite in his next inspection report, and concluded that "no progress has been made in reducing dust concentrations in the dry mill to an acceptable level and that, indeed, the dust concentrations had increased substantially over those in the past." The following year—the same month Grace bought out Zonolite—Wake found dust concentrations at more than fifteen times the limit set by the Public Health Service.

Grace did follow one of Wake's recommendations: in 1964 the corporation installed a huge exhaust fan in the dry mill. Dust levels in the dry mill—though still exceeding acceptable standards even in those days—nonetheless dropped dramatically. Unfortunately the fan vented out into the shop yard where the maintenance crew was stationed, exposing a whole new set of workers to elevated levels of asbestos-contaminated dust. It would take four years for Grace to add a length of pipe onto that exhaust vent and direct the stack up and away from their employees.

In the spring of 1964, Wake noted the new fan, but lamented, "it is unfortunate that the good work that has been done in the ventilation system is reduced by extremely poor housekeeping." Broken screens, leaky boxes, and dusty rafters all kept dust levels in some areas at nearly twelve times the Public Health Service limit.

Numerous people—including Grace's own safety officer, Peter Kostic—recommended that men working as dry mill sweepers be given an alternative to cleaning with push brooms and high-pressure air hoses that sent clouds of dust whirling in the air, but the company never got around to making a change.

Thirty years later, lawyers would grill Earl Lovick about the details of these reports. Why didn't Zonolite and Grace take the simple steps of improving maintenance and stepping up their housekeeping efforts? Lovick insists they did, yet Wake continued to find ill-fitting rubber connectors, missing screens, holes either punched in pipes by rocks or cut by miners so they could reach in and remove obstructions. Wake recommended that the company invest in a portable vacuum system, which Lovick says Grace tried without success. In addition to a bunch of minor hitches, the managers just couldn't figure out what to do with that much dust. Within a year of Lovick's deposition he would be dead, the only one of the three managers present at that first meeting with Wake not to die because of asbestos. Bleich died in 1968 of asbestos-inspired lung cancer, Baker in 1983 of asbestosis proper.

The damage done to these men's lungs by the asbestos Wake documented was not just theoretical but a reality that began with Zonolite's first series of chest X rays in 1959, and continued throughout Grace's ownership until the mine's closure in 1990. That first series, which Zonolite undertook in order to get a baseline for the amount of lung disease among the men, revealed that of 130 employees, 48 had "abnormal" chests—a catchall phrase that included emphysema, tuberculosis, "metallic objects," and old bone breaks and fractures, as well as asbestos-related changes. Rudolph Engle, a Zonolite miner for fourteen years, would die the following year. He was designated, in retrospect, to be the first documented death of asbestos-related disease from the mine at Libby. Grace instituted its own annual X-ray program in 1964. Respiratory function tests taken by 140 men that year "showed that their respiratory function was below standard, that a serious hazard from Pneumoconiosis (lung condition resulting from inhalation of dust particles) exists to employees at Libby." One out of four employees had "lung conditions which might be the start of asbestosis" in 1966. The 1969 X rays indicated that 65 percent of employees who had worked at the mine for twenty years or more had some form of asbestos-related lung disease. Grace commissioned an external study in 1978 that listed 44 out of 205 men as having either asbestos disease or possible asbestos disease. The list of those afflicted included Earl Lovick and Chief Engineer Ray Kujawa.

Another list generated that year reads like the lab report of a mad scientist: Floyd Cole, age forty-eight, employed since 1949. His disease is moderate, first picked up by X rays in 1959. Tom DeShazer, age sixty, employed since 1946. His lungs are severe, the changes first seen in 1964. Fifty-six-year-old Willis Fields also started working for the mine in 1946, with a minor case of lung disease first detected in 1966. Fifteen men are on that list. The author of the memo, manager Bob Oliverio, notes that this is "interesting information." Lloyd Fiscus, age fifty-five, employed by Grace in 1972, moderate disease first detected in 1978. Ed Hendrickson, thirty-six, moderate disease after eighteen years of employment. Morissa Kair, age fifty-nine, with severely damaged lungs, having spent twenty-five years at the mine.

Many of the men, or their surviving family members, say they were never told that they were developing lung disease. In a 1975 letter, Lovick noted that local doctors had not been passing this information along to the miners, and suggested that the company begin informing the men of their medical conditions directly. Spokesperson Alan Stringer says this was the practice during his time at the mine, from 1981 to the facility's closure in 1990. "I can't attest to what was done before I came there," he says. "I can tell you emphatically in the time frame I was there that if there was any abnormality or any change between one year and the next year on a person's X ray, he was told specifically by the manager of that operation."

But Dr. Brad Black, now in charge of Libby's Center for Asbestos Related Disease, says that asbestos-related changes happen so slowly, a change from year to year often isn't sufficient to render any kind of diagnosis. The doctors, he says, probably didn't understand the significance of minor changes on their patients' X rays. "If you were a worker at W.R. Grace, and you had an X ray every year and you had a lung function test, you know you look at the chest X ray and they [Grace] contract one person to read them. But about every four or five years they'd change that person. Because each year there might be a little change, they may say, 'Very slight change in scarring.' Very slight change. Their medical officer for W.R. Grace would review all these and then give the report to the patient, and they'd say basically no change in the X ray this year. Because he'd interpret it as a slight change, minimal change, as basically the same, right? Okay. And your breathing test—breathing tests vary. So you get a little change here. So anyway you add that up over five to ten years, you see what I'm saying? If you looked at it here and then looked at it eight to ten years later, it's a striking change. Unless you followed that patient and that X ray, you wouldn't know what was going on."

Former union president Bob Wilkins says this was his experience exactly. "We'd go down to the hospital here, and the only results that we'd ever get, if we ever got anything at all, would be a letter from Grace in Cambridge," he says. "And he would give us a statement to the effect that there was no change from the year before. We didn't know what the hell the year before was either. So we had no idea really of what was taking place."

Since no one outside of the corporation was looking at the big picture—not in terms of each man's life over the span of years or at the workforce as a whole—few people noticed anything amiss, and no one told the patients.

One didn't need to be a radiologist to know that something was wrong with some of the men. During his twenty-five years at Grace's mine, Bob Wilkins was elected union job steward and treasurer. He was entrusted three times with the Local 361's presidency, and now he is designated as the keeper of a dead man's memory. "You ask Bob Wilkins about the last days of Tom Craver," I'm told several times. So I do.

Craver was a supervisor, Wilkins tells me. He worked at the screening plant by the river, where vermiculite was separated by size into five different grades. "He got into real bad, bad shape," Wilkins begins. "He got so that he couldn't hardly walk across the floor without stopping to breathe, and he was gasping for air. And I seen this one day, and I seen it several times. But this one time, it really upset me because he worked with other people, and occasionally his job would have to be riding the man-lift up to the sixth floor. Man-lift. You know what a man-lift is? It's like a conveyor belt with steps on it. And you step on this and you have handholds above you and you hold onto that and it takes you up to whatever floor you want.

"He had occasion to go up there to check screens or something, and the man wasn't capable. He couldn't do that job safely was the problem. I got really concerned about it, and I called Lovick. I said, 'What in the hell you got this guy still working here for?' I said,

'He's endangering his life and the people that's working with him, because if he ever falls into one of them machines, or falls and gets hung up on that man-lift, we could injure someone else trying to help him.' I said, 'The guy's not physically able to work any longer. I want you to make a note of this, that I'm telling you right now, so that if something happens, I want a record made of this.'"

Soon after, Lovick came by the screening plant one afternoon and took Tom Craver home. He died not much later, in 1977.

Over the years, men judged to be ill appear to have been moved to less hazardous jobs—not for their protection, but to keep them working. In 1968, Grace safety officer Peter Kostic speculated that if Grace could keep sick workers from being exposed to more dust, "chances are that we may be able to keep them on the job until they retire, thus precluding the high cost of total disability."

Ben Wake recommended time and again that workers be provided with respirators temporarily, while Zonolite and later Grace got the dust problem under control. In fact, Lovick testified, respirators were not only provided, they were required from 1954 on. The company kept two bins just outside the dry mill—one filled with clean respirators, from which the men could pick out a new one every time their filter clogged up, and one for the dirty respirators. It was a practice Grace continued, even as officials acknowledged the respirators' shortcomings as dust control policy. Even Safety Officer Kostic wrote, "respirators should not be considered a substitute for proper engineering controls. Respirators are fine for short periods of time, but to get a man to wear one eight hours a day is next to impossible." Especially when, as Lovick admitted in court, the miners were not told until 1979 why wearing the respirators was imperative.

Grace officials moved slowly toward closing the dusty dry mill—a step that was eleven years in the making, forty-four years after the medical community first recommended that industry phase out dry asbestos processing. Why did it take so long? As Stringer told me, there's no one left alive to ask this question of. But a 1965 interoffice memo from Joseph Kelley, a Chicago executive left over from the old Zonolite days, sheds some light on the matter. He wrote, "the second important decision made at Libby was that we would move as fast as possible to eliminate the dry mill. This has been our plan all along but because of our balance problem we could not see the light as to when this could be done." Grace distributed $20.6 million in profits to its shareholders that year, according to court records. The process was sped up when the State of Montana cited Grace for air pollution violations in 1969. The citations apparently were a serious matter. According to a 1975 internal performance report, "If Zonolite had not been actively working to solve these pollution problems at Libby, a forced shutdown of the facilities would have occurred in 1972." Grace requested, and was granted, a series of extensions to meet the provisions of the law, but doing so was costly: the company spent $6.75 million to build a ten-story wet mill, a dam for the tailings pond, and a new dust collection system and screening plant at the loading station on the river, among other improvements. Lincoln County commissioners helped take the edge off by issuing $6 million in revenue bonds, which allowed Grace to pay for the project at a lower interest rate than it would have obtained in the private bond market.

The new mill came online in 1974. Two men died from Grace's dust that year: Gayla and Eva's father, Perley Vatland, and a miner named Lilas "Shorty" Welch.

The case of Shorty Welch nearly blew Grace's secret dust problem into the public's eye, a situation that was averted only by quick action on the part of a lawyer for Grace's insurance company. Shorty went to work at the Libby mine in 1949, starting out as most of the men did in the dry mill. He was promoted to work in the on-site warehouse in 1956, and was misdiagnosed with silicosis three years later. Welch continued to work for Grace until 1966, when he filed for disability. Initially, Grace execs decided to dodge responsibility. In a series of letters and memos between Grace and its insurance company, officials plotted to defend themselves by claiming Welch did not have asbestosis proper, and that if he did, it was contracted before the State of Montana adopted its Industrial Disease Act, and furthermore that asbestosis was not added to the

list of compensable diseases until 1965. If Welch contracted asbestosis as a result of his work at Grace, they reasoned, it must have
happened in the dry mill—way before 1965. His case was headed
for a workers' comp hearing—it would have been the first among
Libby miners—when Grace's insurance lawyer intervened.

Four days before the hearing began, Maryland Casualty Company attorney S. Y. Larrick wrote an eight-page letter strongly urg-
ing Grace to settle the case. Larrick started out by noting that

> it might appear to others that the action taken by insured to
> correct the situation which was present, might not to the unbiased
> observer, appear to have been either extremely effective, or
> quickly performed. ... I would hesitate to allow in evidence the
> State Board reports if it is possible to keep them out of the hands
> of the Industrial Accident Board, and through it, the general
> public. While I have not researched the problem, it has even
> occurred to me that insured's inability to curb the problem at the
> State Board's recommendations through the years, might alleged
> to have constituted willful and wanton conduct on its part, with
> whatever complications that particular charge might carry with it.

Larrick punched a hole in Grace's theory that Shorty's asbestosis
could only have been due to working in the dry mill, pointing out
that the mill exhaust vented into a nearby yard next to the warehouse where Welch worked—a situation criticized over the years
by both Ben Wake and Libby's union officials. Welch, he wrote,
"may well have suffered 'an injurious exposure' as that term may
be defined in the Occupational Disease Act, at most every point
he was employed, including the warehouse." Furthermore, Larrick
reported that the insurance company's own expert witness had
said he would have to support Welch's claim were he to testify.

Acting swiftly, Grace managed to halt the hearing halfway, after
Welch had begun to make his case, but before Grace was forced to
produce any damaging evidence. Nevertheless the company knew
the potential fallout from Shorty's case could be far-reaching. "The
implications of the case are apparent. A record has now been made
that there is danger of asbestosis in our operation," Grace official
Charles Dugan wrote. "Unfortunately, however, we know that

there is a potentially large group of employees who may already have the beginnings of the disease so that eventual liability cannot be readily forecast. Undoubtedly we will be required to take further and more expensive measures for limiting the exposure.

"Also unmentioned in these discussions was any question of moral obligation apart from legal liability."

IN 1976, GRACE HIRED ITS first on-site industrial hygienist to work at the Libby mine. Randy Geiger, then an enthusiastic young man from a tiny town in eastern Montana with the ink practically still drying on his diploma from Montana Tech, recalls being excited about the challenges Grace laid before him. "They had the asbestos problem and they knew that they had a problem. They had people at Cambridge, at the corporate headquarters, but they didn't have anybody on-site. I was the first engineer, industrial hygiene. And basically I set up an industrial hygiene program and sampling for asbestos."

Geiger started working for Grace just as the kinks were worked out of the new dry mill, and he reported in memo after memo the dramatic drop in asbestos fiber counts. Men in the dry mill, for instance, were still breathing air with as many as 85 asbestos fibers per milliliter of air in 1973. Four years later, Geiger found the asbestos levels dropping monthly in the new wet mill, down to .12 fibers/ml that spring. A report from Grace's insurance company seconds these findings: "Airborne fiber counts in the range of 20 to 60 fibers/cc were common before 1974," wrote Richard Dolliver, a regional manager for Maryland Casualty, who noted that the range dropped initially to between 1 and 10 fibers per cubic centimeter of air, and even further in some areas. "Some personnel exposures still exceeded 2.0 fibers/cc and about 30 percent are .5 fibers and above."

This was good news for Grace officials, who had been weighing the costs of meeting a proposed new standard of .5 fibers/ml. "We may now be able to operate without additional pollution control at the proposed .5 fiber limit," Geiger said.

Although these numbers represented dramatic improvements, three facts offset the success. First, the new lower fiber limits still exposed workers to enough asbestos to make them sick. Second, the standard method used to detect and count the fibers—phase contrast microscopy—missed literally thousands of asbestos fibers in any given sample—a fact not even the EPA would figure out until twenty years later. And third, a friendly Grace researcher named Julie Yang had developed her own way of counting fibers, and so ended up with counts far lower than other researchers found.

"If you don't have any training, everything looks like a fiber because it looks like a line under the microscope," she tells me in a telephone interview. "If you use the standard counting, anything that looks like a line, you count it. You may count 15 out of your field." Yang says she examined each sample more closely, twisted it around to get the full picture, and was more accurately able to distinguish asbestos fibers from everything else under her microscope. "So if we use our—we call it our way of counting—we probably could get 10 or 8, something like that. And then we look at the whole thing with an electron microscope to see which one is exactly the fiber. We have a lot of data, so that's why we use our method and nobody disputes it."

Randy Geiger has one other claim to fame in Libby. Sometime around 1980, mine manager Bill McCaig okayed the use of mine tailings to pave a running track for the local high school. "It was kind of a political thing, it was kind of a big deal to be on the school board. He was trying to be popular in the school district. So for some reason he gave them a bunch of tailings," Geiger says.

"I called him. I said, 'Bill, that probably wasn't the smartest thing you ever did.'

"'Well ... it's just like cinders; they can run on it.'

"'But it's got asbestos in it!'"

Geiger says he was flabbergasted. So Geiger put air samplers on himself and his wife, Heather (daughter of Dr. MacKenzie, who misdiagnosed Gayla Benefield's father with a nonexistent heart problem), and they went for a run. They kicked up asbestos fibers at .14 and .22 fibers/cc. "Fiber concentrations were surprisingly high considering the sampling conditions," Geiger reported to McCaig in a 1981 memo. "It is my opinion that short-term concentrations as high as 1.0 f/cc could result when the track is in a well-used condition and is being used by a large number of people."

Geiger, who now lives with his family in a small town near Bozeman, Montana, says he remembers the tailings being used on the track only that one time. But another Grace memo reports the track had been paved with mine tailings repeatedly beginning in the early 1970s. After the Geigers' track-and-field experiment, Grace paid to pave over the tailings. In the summer of 2001 the EPA would have to excavate the track to a depth of a foot and a half to dig out all the asbestos—a fact that would irritate the business community to distraction when the beginning of the fall football season had to be postponed.

The Libby managers in 1977 raised the question of installing showers and providing the miners with uniforms, saying, "We do not have adequate locker and toilet facilities at Libby at this time." Former union president Bob Wilkins recalls there was one shower stall for all the men, located in the new wet mill. "One shower for the mine crew, the mill crew, the welding shop, construction shop, garage. I don't know if anyone ever used the shower for showering at all," he says. After each shift the company bused its men from the mine site back downtown, so there wasn't time even if someone was inclined to rinse off. "You had like fifteen minutes from the time you were off shift. They allowed you like fifteen minutes to put away your tools, get back to your department, put away your tools, wash up, and get ready to go home. You had fifteen minutes.

"You couldn't do it. It was impossible."

Five years later the company decided against spending an extra $373,000 on showers, uniforms, and paid overtime—the cost of giving miners the chance to clean the dust off their bodies before heading home to their families. That year, 1982, Grace set a record for profits, issuing $130.9 million to shareholders, a number that would increase in 1997 to $467.9 million, according to information culled from court records and Grace's 2000 annual report. It was 1984, more than twenty years after Grace bought the mine, when employees were issued coveralls.

Nineteen seventy-nine was a watershed year. It started out inno-
cently enough. A train derailment took out Grace's loading facility by the river, so union president Bob Wilkins found himself and
his shipping department working out of the old expansion plant
downtown by the ball fields—where Les Skramstad and crew conducted their "asbestos project" two decades earlier—when the federal Mine Safety and Health Administration came by to do an
inspection. Wilkins then found out what was in the dust he'd been
breathing for thirteen years. There was nothing unusual about the
inspection, he says. MSHA sent inspectors out three or four times
a year. This particular one stayed for three days, and he and
Wilkins became friendly. "He was telling me about his job and how
many places he'd been to in the states, the type of mines he'd
worked in, and so forth. And he mentioned copper mines in Arizona, New Mexico, and Colorado and the dangers that were involved there with the asbestos and the type of dust that they had.

"And I just mentioned to him, I said, 'We're kind of fortunate
here we don't have asbestos to worry with, we have—'

"He says, 'You don't?'

"And I said, 'No, we have tremolite.'" Wilkins says Grace had
told the union it was planning to start an antismoking program,
and as part of that had begun dropping the word "tremolite." "Asbestos," he says, was not part of the new vocabulary.

"So I told the inspector, I said, 'Well, we're fortunate that we
don't have an asbestos problem, we have tremolite.' And he looked
at me kind of odd, and he said, 'Well, just a second.' And he goes
over to his government bag and he brings this book back; it has all
the different classifications of different dust and whatever. It's
kinda like the Bible; in fact it's about the size of the Bible. So he
turns to 'asbestos' and 'tremolite' was the number one. ... Asbestos
had four classifications—tremolite was number one."

Wilkins worked out his shift, then stopped by Grace headquarters on Mineral Avenue to drop off that day's shipping orders. Earl
Lovick was there, so Wilkins stepped in to the boss's office.

"I walked in and said, 'Earl, we got a problem.'

"And he said, 'What kind of problem?'

"And I said, 'Well, for a hell of a long time you've been telling us that we've got a nuisance dust.'

"He said, 'Yeah, that's right.'

"I said, 'Here lately you've been dropping the word "tremolite."'

"'Yeah,' he said, 'that's what we work with.'

"I said, 'Why in the hell didn't you go a step further and tell us it contained asbestos and one of the worst types of asbestos in the classifications?" Wilkins is from Tennessee and as he becomes angry with the telling, the South comes out in his voice.

"He kinda threw up his hands and said, 'Bob, I thought everybody knew that.' And I come unglued then, and I told him there wasn't a guy on that damned hill up there was a dust engineer. And I questioned if anyone up there knew the definition of 'tremolite,' what the hell it was in the dust. We didn't have any clue as to the classifications, but I told him, I said, 'You can bet your ass when the next union meeting comes around, everybody's going to know about it.' And from that time on, whenever anyone talked to me about dust—union members, non-union members—anyone, I explained to them exactly what tremolite was and how dangerous it was. And I also told employees, union members, anyone else that they had already been exposed to it for a number of years. They could make their choice as to whatever they wanted to do. Some left and went to other jobs. Some stayed on."

Wilkins stayed on, rationalizing that he'd already been exposed to Grace's asbestos for thirteen years, and that he was in a far less dusty position than he had been in the past. Plus, he thought, maybe the asbestos situation was not so bad after all. He explains that when he complained to other managers, their actions spoke louder than their words: "I was told by both of those people it was no more than a nuisance dust, it was no more harmful to you than farm dust. ... While they were telling me this, they were standing right alongside me breathing the same air that I was. It's kinda hard to feel that a guy's lying to you when he's standing right beside you, breathing the same air for eight hours a day."

When he was thinking of retiring in 1988, Wilkins drove over to see Dr. Alan Whitehouse, a pulmonologist in Spokane who treats many of Libby's asbestos patients, who told him he had pleural plaquing, but that it wasn't necessarily fatal. "He did tell me that the way these things work, as years go on they can produce a problem. So when I left his office, I felt real good. I felt that I had been able to work there and escape without any bad side effects. I felt real great when I left his office. I got out of there. I felt home free."

He wasn't. Wilkins is on oxygen now, his life limited by his lung capacity most days to puttering around the neat second-story apartment where he lives downtown next to the river. A bowl full of Tootsie Pops sitting next to the "No Smoking" sign on the coffee table attests to his great-grandsons' presence in his life, and while the whole family still goes camping on occasion, it's hard for Wilkins. "My sons come up. They're real nice about that. They help set up the camp for me, they do most of it. All's I do is just sit there and boss."*

GRACE IMPOSED A ban on smoking on company property in the summer of 1979. The company estimated that nearly 80 percent of the men smoked, and so the new policy was not a popular one. It was, however, a long time in the making. A renowned asbestos expert, Dr. Irving Selikoff of Mt. Sinai Hospital in New York, had published in 1968 a groundbreaking study on the synergistic effects of smoking and asbestos exposure in the *Journal of the American Medical Association*. Among Selikoff's study group of asbestos insulation workers, none of the nonsmokers died of lung cancer. Of the 283 smokers, for which models predicted three lung cancer deaths, Selikoff recorded twenty-four such deaths. He concluded that "asbestos workers who smoke have about 92 times the risk of dying of bronchogenic carcinoma as men who neither work with asbestos nor smoke cigarettes. We conclude that asbestos exposure should be minimized, that asbestos workers who do not smoke should never start, and that those now smoking should stop immediately." With this study in hand, Grace officials began talking amongst themselves about a smoking ban in Libby by 1969. While

---

*Wilkins died of asbestos-related causes on November 10, 2002.

it was another decade before they got around to doing anything about it, Lovick took on the matter himself. A smoker, Lovick told lawyers he had plaque peeled from his lungs in 1971 or 1972. His doctor told him it was related to asbestos exposure, so he quit smoking and became an antismoking demagogue.

"I told many, many people … what they were doing to their health by their smoking," he said. "And you might say that some of them I begged that they quit smoking." Once again, however, Lovick said he did not tell his workers about the asbestos or about Selikoff's study. "I just told them not to smoke basically." And when they didn't listen, he was once again frustrated. "And for all practical purposes I might have been just as well been talking to the wall because it had no effect."

By the late 1970s, even an outsider would notice things weren't all well at Grace's Zonolite division. The mine weathered its first strike—over wages and benefits—in 1978. This was followed by a series of temporary shutdowns and layoffs through the early 1980s, ostensibly to "reduce inventories that have built up due to the sagging construction market," the local *Western News* reported. Part of that equation, however, was a decision by one of Grace's largest customers, the O.M. Scott Company (known for its lawn care and gardening products), to stop using Libby vermiculite after its Ohio workers began getting sick. One shutdown occurred just after the lumber mill, the old J. Neils plant (which had switched owners several times over the years), announced it would be closing for good. Libby's economy was headed for hard times.

Grace began to consider the possibility that it would have to close the Libby mine. In a long 1977 memo on possible regulatory scenarios and subsequent effects on the mine's profitability, Grace executive vice president E. S. Wood laid out the worst case: "Our best estimate is that a 1 f/ml standard for Libby would require 3.6 million dollars of additional capital. A tightening of OSHA [Occupational Safety and Health Administration] regulations covering our expanding plants to a level of .1 f/ml would require 6 million dollars of additional capital." Such standards, he wrote, "would make it uneconomical to continue operating Libby." By

1990 the threat of tightened regulations, coupled with the loss of the Scott Company business and a dramatic decrease in the market for asbestos-containing products, forced the end. Grace shut down the Libby mine. Grace safety director Harry Eschenbach told lawyers at a 1997 deposition that the closure had been in the works for nearly a decade. In the mid-1980s, he says, "there started to be this, I guess, overly strong concern about asbestos, far beyond what any scientific approach would indicate.

"Competitors made that allegation, that there was asbestos with the Libby vermiculite. And whether it was true or not, the asbestos phobia was strong enough so that it dramatically affected the demand for Libby vermiculite."

Four years after the closure, the *Western News* spoke with a bitter Alan Stringer, reporting that "when it was shut down, the mine still had 50 million tons of proven reserves, which could have provided another 55 years of operation at the peak level—200,000 tons per year—of shipments.

"'A viable use for a mineral has been eliminated,' said Stringer. 'In today's regulatory climate it will never be permitted again.'"

Although this story mentions in passing that Libby vermiculite was contaminated with "a few parts per million asbestos," and although the obituary pages by then were full of miners dying of asbestos-related disease, the scope of Libby's sickness remained secret, buried with vermiculite in the gardens and forgotten in the walls of attics.

Exiled

Lerah Parker has a photo album to beat them all. She and her husband, Mel, starting taking pictures of their Raintree Nursery business when they bought the property by the Kootenai River at its juncture with Rainy Creek in 1993. They'd been in the business for seven years already, but had outgrown their old 5-acre plot across town. Relative newcomers to Libby—Mel grew up in Canada, Lerah in eastern Montana—they had little reason to suspect that the dirt from which they planned to cultivate life would harbor death.

This new piece of land, 21 acres formerly owned by the W.R. Grace corporation, was barren to start with. That first year, there was not a tree or a blade of grass on the place, Lerah tells me. In six years, she and Mel transformed the place.

"We had almost every nursery plant that was native to this area growing on our property. We had how many fruit trees in the orchard. We were trying every variety of fruit tree, all the way from walnuts to peach trees to apricots to specialized pears. If they could adapt to our property, then we could go ahead and sell them and know they would do well in Libby. If they didn't adapt to our property after three or four years, then they weren't hardy enough to sell to the public. ...

"It was landscaped in such a way, like we had almost 102 roses, different types of roses on the property, and we had a bark path with different flowers, all the different colors of mums."

They grew organically certified herbs in raised beds, Echinacea seedlings, and tree seedlings—300,000 annually—for timber companies and the U.S. Forest Service's reforestation projects. They cultivated flowers for their floral shop downtown and ran a landscaping business out of a long shed that came with the property, renting out space in the shed during the off-season for RV and boat storage. In the tunnels where Grace once used conveyor belts to haul ore out of the long storage shed and across the river, Lerah had started a mushroom-growing project.

"In Japan the Reishi mushroom is considered a cure for some forms of cancer. So when they had this conveyor system inside the tunnels there, they took the conveyors out, but they left the vermiculite on the ground," Mel explains. "All that material was just vermiculite that hadn't been expanded, but had fallen off the belts. So what we did was we took our buckets and they were what, 4-gallon buckets? And we scooped it up with shovels and filled the buckets up with vermiculite because it's an excellent medium for growing Reishi mushrooms. It's got a very good ability to retain water. It doesn't have any nutrients in it but we didn't need it anyway. What we did is, we went out into the woods and cut alder trees down and that was for the mushrooms.

"We drilled fourteen holes in each one of the logs, and that portion that was above the level of the vermiculite in the buckets, we had plugs—wood plugs, wooden dowels? And they were like she said; they were inoculated with spawn and we put those in the logs, and we put them in the buckets. They just started growing and pretty soon the mushrooms would come out the sides of the logs. Then we would harvest the mushrooms."

Lerah chimes in: "Well we got our first crop in, we inoculated in May of '99, and they were growing very well. We were just coming online to start cultivating and the EPA came in and threw the whole project out. Everything. They just went in there and threw everything out, trashed it all."

The Parkers built a home on their property and lived there. They baby-sat their four grandchildren after school and the kids practically lived there with them in the summers. They erected greenhouses and maintained a road down to the river so the public could picnic and fish. One of the local churches held sunrise services on the Parkers' land as it had for forty-two years. It was, Lerah tells me, a special place to a lot of people in Libby.

Now it's all gone.

The land is there, barren as it ever was now that the bulldozers have worked on it for two years. Lerah's photos show this too: the roof taken off their house; all their possessions—clothing, television, everything—still inside; the heavy machinery crushing it all to smithereens. Now it is encircled by a series of chain-link fences behind which moon-suited government contractors are doing their best to dig up all of W.R. Grace's asbestos, making it safe for the Parker family to live there again.

Both the Parkers have evidence of asbestos scarring in their lungs after a mere six years spent on the property. Lerah's is more pronounced; she coughs already, and Spokane doctor Alan Whitehouse has told her she can expect her symptoms to get markedly worse in the next few years. But they're more concerned for their grandkids.

"One of the areas they really called a high hit on, that had a high percentage of asbestos in it, was right on the front lawn," Mel says. "About 4 feet away from the swing set, and that's where the grandkids played." A granddaughter, Lerah adds, was exposed almost daily from the time she was six months old. A grandson probably got a good dose too: he loved to dig in the dirt. "Jeffrey had a bulldozer and he would play in that stuff all the time with his little bulldozer. He just loved playing in the dirt. I planted marigolds all along the front of the house, and he took his bulldozer out there and dozed them all up and laid 'em nice and neat in a pile."

The Parkers live in town now, in a home leased for them by the government, making ends meet with a $1,900 monthly stipend from the feds. They're not too bad off financially: they had managed to pay off every bit of debt they had on their business (except for six months left on a truck loan) just before the EPA came in and took it all away. Nevertheless, they have nothing but good things to say about the agency's team leader, Paul Peronard, and only disgust for Grace. They entered what they thought were negotiations with the company to settle the matter, but emerged from those talks bitter.

"It was a big joke to them," Lerah says. "A big joke."

"They wanted to take all the contaminated soil—we had 20 acres, all right? They wanted to take 5 acres where the long shed was and bring all the contaminated soil into that and make that a deed-restricted area," Mel says. No compensation for those 5 acres either. "Grace wouldn't give us any liability. They wouldn't indemnify us—you know, for example, if you were a customer of ours and you had your boat stored there. And unless the EPA allowed Grace to do the cleanup, then the contract would be void. There was all kinds of things that Grace was wanting us to do, but they weren't really going to do anything for us."

"They made an appointment with us; they came forty-five minutes late," Lerah says. "Didn't even look at our property. Had an offer on the table with a set amount and that was it. Tried to show him the property; he had no interest in anything that we had going on. Absolutely none. Told him about the Reishi project—he laughed. It was just a big joke to those people. They had a set amount when they walked in the door, and if we didn't like it, great. They said, 'Go back and think it over' and they'll meet with us in a couple more weeks. We met with them two weeks later and his attitude didn't change. He said ..."

Mel interrupts. "He said, 'We'll see you folks in court in five to seven years.'"

FIVE

Anatomy of Silence

FOR SOMEONE WHO HAS just been accused, essentially, of being a Good German, Brad Black responds with surprisingly good humor. While he now runs Libby's Center for Asbestos Related Diseases (CARD), Dr. Black was once a pediatrician. I've just told him that Gayla Benefield faults him for hiding behind his young clientele in the 1970s and 1980s, while the adults were dying. He laughs, a little awkwardly. Gayla has become a friend, and he's learned to take her acerbic wit as an indication of affection. "I don't think she meant that I purposely hid behind it. I didn't purposely hide behind it. I was just in it. I didn't have any direct involvement with people who were affected by asbestosis.

"We didn't know, see, at that time, we had no idea what exposures were occurring with kids."

Black is an Indiana native, son of an NBA ballplayer whose lanky frame is concealed behind a lab coat until he props his legs on top of his desk. He moved to Libby in 1977 when some medical school buddies asked if he'd like to start a clinic with them. He agreed, and they set up shop in a two-story house in a residential neighborhood near downtown. Black was the pediatrician, Richard Irons the internist, Bruce Hardy the general practitioner. Hardy lasted only a couple of years—Libby's climate was too hard on his allergies. Irons, too, left within a decade. He figured out early on that something was wrong at the mine, and spent most of his Libby years banging his head against Grace's corporate wall of silence. Now only Black is left.

The CARD clinic is a rather humble setting for treating what an EPA official has termed "the worst industrial accident in U.S. history." The building is little more than a glorified double-wide trailer plopped down in a vacant lot kitty-corner from Libby's St. Johns Lutheran Hospital. The clinic runs, for now, on portions of the $250,000 Grace agreed to donate annually to the town's medical community. In taking this job, Black is paying some long-unsettled dues.

"The perception at least from my end was that there were people, agencies, involved, and various things going on in the '80s were bringing [Grace] in line with regulations that would protect workers," he says. "I guess the thing that you learn from that is the agencies have to be held accountable."

Black is reluctant to implicate his fellow doctors, the half-dozen or so men who constituted Libby's medical community through the 1960s and 1970s. While some clearly knew their patients were being made sick by something at the mine, Black insists hindsight is simply too convenient. But the relationship between Grace and the doctors is a curious one, and to understand it it's helpful to know a little about the history of asbestos itself.

Asbestos was once thought to be the flameproof hair of an amphibian, a salamander that lived in fire. Its history dates back to 3000 B.C., when Egyptians wove asbestos fibers into burial cloth and Romans wrapped those bound for cremation in asbestos fabric to hold the ashes together. Another story is that Charlemagne, the eighth-century king of the Franks, threw an asbestos tablecloth on the fireplace after dinner—both to clean it and to impress his guests.

Asbestos is a silicate, made up of silicon and oxygen. As an element, silicon is second in abundance only to oxygen, with which it readily combines to form silicon dioxide, or silica. Silica tends to crystallize, with lovely results: quartz, jasper, agate. There are six recognized varieties of asbestos, all characterized by their fibrous form. And while the silicates have long been known to cause silicosis among miners, it was not until the early 1900s that scientists and doctors began to recognize asbestosis as a distinct disease—primarily because it wasn't until the Industrial Revolution that asbestos was mined on a large scale. The first reported cases of asbestosis occurred around the turn of the century; the "Lady Inspectors" who worked the British textile industry noted respiratory disease among the employees. British doctor Murray Montague reported a case to his government in 1907.

For the next twenty-three years or so, scientists would busy themselves debating whether asbestosis was a separate disease from silicosis, recording its symptoms and guessing at methods for diagnosis. In 1930, researchers noted that while the effects of asbestos can appear early in the lungs, there is a long latency period—ten to forty years—before the disease manifests. Two researchers writing in the *Journal of the American Medical Association* (*JAMA*) in that year related finding asbestos fibers in the lungs of a couple of millworkers who died of unrelated causes, both with less than five years working in the industry. An editorial in *JAMA* that same year noted the latency period of the disease in an asbestos miner who died from it—thirty-two years for the man in question—and acknowledged that asbestosis can lead to heart problems. Most of it is dry reading, necessarily narrow in scope. But in 1930, two British researchers reporting to Parliament laid out the entire problem, from the geology of asbestos to the disease's pathology and beyond.

> It is helpful to visualize fibrosis of the lungs as it occurs in asbestos workers as the slow growth of fibrous tissue (scar tissue) between the air cells of the lung wherever the inhaled dust comes to rest. While new fibrous tissue is being laid down like a spider's web, that deposited earlier gradually contracts. This fibrous tissue is not only useless as a substitute for the air cells, but with continued inhalation of the causative dust, by its invasion of new territory and consolidation of that already occupied, it gradually, and literally, strangles the essential tissues of the lungs.
>
> In common with other essential organs of the body the lungs have a large reserve of tissue for use in emergencies and to permit a diminution of functional capacity due to advancing age or disease. For this reason ... it is only when the fibrosis progresses to the extent of obliterating this reserve that undue shortness of breath on any effort draws the worker's attention to the fact that his health is not what it should be.
>
> From this point the progress of the disease is more rapid, since it is now encroaching on the remaining sound tissue of the lungs, already only just sufficient to maintain him in his daily activities.

The second half of the presentation is devoted to prevention. The researchers found that in textile mills, those people exposed to less dust take a longer time to develop asbestosis. "A further point of great practical importance emerges, namely, that in order to prevent the full development of the disease among asbestos workers within the space of an average working lifetime, it is necessary to reduce the concentrations of dust in the air. ..." Workers should be educated so as to have "a sane appreciation of the risk and [as] to his personal responsibility in the prevention and suppression of dust." And while respirators provide some protection, they "can only be recommended as a second line of defense and not in substitution for other preventive measures specifically directed to the control of dust. ..."

The British researchers ended their report with a set of recommendations, including their opinion that industries dealing in asbestos ought to phase out dry processing methods in favor of using water to cut down on dust. It would take another forty-four years for Grace to close Libby's dry mill.

The research continued. A minor breakthrough occurred when researchers realized they could see asbestos fibers in the sputum of textile workers. Pictures accompanying a 1932 report in the *Journal of Pathology* show a delicate pattern of radially arranged fiber clumps, an abstract daisy print that turned out to "indicate merely that asbestos dust has been inhaled into the lung and has remained there for a certain length of time." By that time, others had noted the presence of fiber clumps in workers' phlegm and drawn similar conclusions. But this article is notable in hindsight for an offhand comment, particularly poignant in regard to Libby: the authors found fiber clumps "in the lungs, post mortem, in a man who lived close to a factory for many years but who had never been inside it." In fact in 1956, Ben Wake included similar information in his report to the mine managers, warning of the potential danger to those living nearby, but Zonolite—and later Grace—never told Libby residents of the risk.

A doctor specializing in tuberculosis wrote in 1933 the first comprehensive guide to diagnosing asbestosis in a clinical setting, via X rays and with post-mortem pathological evidence. Dr. Philip Ellman concluded in the *Journal of Industrial Hygiene* that "pulmonary asbestosis, once established, is a progressive disease with a bad prognosis; its treatment can only be symptomatic." Seventy years later, this statement is chillingly accurate. There is no cure for asbestosis. If you have it, you're almost certainly going to die of it—unless, as Gayla Benefield is fond of saying, "you get smacked by a truck first."

Meanwhile, doctors began noticing an unusual number of cancer cases in their asbestos patients. At first scientists considered the connection merely an interesting coincidence. But by 1949, even the skeptics at *JAMA* had to admit the evidence had become convincing: in the process of dissecting dead asbestosis victims, British doctors had found a significantly high occurrence of lung cancer: 13.2 percent of 235 asbestos dead, to be precise. The normal rate would have been something more like 1 percent. *JAMA* noted that while men generally tended to contract lung cancer more than women, the rates among asbestos victims were less disparate, indicating that something in the asbestos industry environment was "equalizing the incidence rate of cancer of the lungs for both sexes." The journal called for increased attention to the likelihood of a causal link between asbestos and cancer, and the medical community obliged. The watershed study—the one generally accepted as conclusive—was published in 1955 by Dr. Richard Doll, who found 11 lung cancers among textile workers where only 0.8 should have occurred.

All kinds of other details would come later. Dr. Irving Selikoff's research would dominate the field in the 1960s, when he laid rest to any niggling doubts about the cancer-asbestos connection. Then there was his groundbreaking study in 1968, which revealed that asbestos workers who smoked were ninety-two times more likely to die from lung cancer than nonsmokers and non–asbestos workers. (Selikoff further shook up the asbestos industry by refusing to stick to pure research. Until his death in 1992, he took on the mantle of advocate, working with unions to strengthen asbestos regulations to protect rank-and-file employees.)

There are lingering questions about how asbestos fibers cause these diseases and whether there is any safe level of exposure. In the 1970s, Grace would still be arguing that tremolite was misclassified as asbestos, and that it had short, fat fibers of the sort less likely to cause asbestosis, unlikely to cause cancer at all. In fact, Grace had plenty of evidence to the contrary, and even had reason to suspect tremolite was more virulent than other forms of asbestos. They did not share this information with local doctors, nor did they reveal it to any of the agencies charged with protecting the health of workers and the public. But the basic facts were all there by 1955: Asbestos causes cancer. Asbestos causes fibrosis. Tremolite is asbestos.

DR. WILLIAM LITTLE was perhaps the only human being outside of the Grace corporation who saw the big picture of disease in Libby. A Scotsman by birth, he moved to Montana in 1958 and set up shop as an "itinerant radiologist," traveling to tiny hospitals up and down the Flathead Valley and beyond. He worked the funky spa town of Hot Springs, the old mission at St. Ignatius, Ronan on the reservation, Polson at the southern tip of Flathead Lake, and Whitefish under the shadow of Big Mountain. He spent a day or two per week in Libby, and vaguely recalls that sometime prior to 1959, he saw his first case of asbestosis in a Zonolite miner. "A patient came into the hospital for maybe a routine chest [X ray] preoperatively, which was done routinely at the time," he told lawyers at a 1997 deposition. "Or he may have come into the hospital sick for some other reason. So I don't really know when it was. It was just one of the men that worked out there showed up and I saw findings that I thought were very indicative of asbestosis." He found this curious and spoke to Earl Lovick about it, indicating it might be worth taking X rays of the mine's entire workforce. "When we first talked, I told him that these findings were strongly suggestive of asbestosis, and I asked, 'Is there asbestos there?' And he said, 'We have been told that there is no significant asbestos fiber in our dust.'

"And I guess at that time I was a little confused because I was almost certain the diagnosis was asbestosis and it had to come from somewhere." Subsequently, he found that Earl meant there was no commercial grade asbestos at the mine. There was, Lovick eventually told Dr. Little, a short-fibered tremolite.

Little recommended that Zonolite X-ray all its miners, and in 1959 the State of Montana gave the company further reason to do so. That year, Montana enacted an occupational disease law, holding companies responsible for work-related injuries and illnesses. The new law was not retroactive, so Libby's management decided they needed to get a record of which employees were already sick—and therefore not covered by the law—in case of future claims. "In order to protect ourselves and place ourselves on record as to the condition of our employees as of the effective date of the law," Lovick wrote, "we instituted a program whereby all of our employees would have x-rays at the local hospital."

Little testified that he helped plan the X-ray program in 1959 and analyzed the results: 48 out of 142 men had abnormal chests. He told Lovick that short of doing biopsies on all these men, a 100 percent–sure diagnosis was not possible. Still, he told the lawyers, the evidence they had after the first battery of X rays was convincing. "To get an absolute diagnosis, I suppose you had to find the asbestos fiber some way if you really were going to prove it. But if you have the hallmarks, all these findings were severe in a lot of cases, very typical, and predominant in our view of the chest. And the place they worked had the asbestos fiber. You add the two together and you come up with a pretty conclusive finding. ...

"We [he and Lovick] talked about the number of cases we were seeing, probably coming from that plant, and that that was a very significant finding that we were seeing."

The chief of staff at Libby's hospital, Dr. James Cairns, outlined a follow-up program for the men with abnormal X rays, a plan that included doing a complete physical exam, including taking each patient's full history, giving him a tuberculin test, taking a sputum sample, and taking more X rays. Little recalled that Grace was to forward the X-ray reports to each worker's family physician, along with the follow-up recommendations. Little, meanwhile, told Lovick he wanted to see the X-ray series continued at least every two years, maybe more often for the men with diseased lungs. Grace instituted an annual program in 1964 and paid the hospital to cover Little's salary for the job. During the two decades Little read Grace's black-and-white film, the results varied little. There was a low of 19 percent abnormals one year, a high of 41 percent another. The average, from 1964 to 1981, counted just under 28 percent of the miners showing evidence of lung disease.

Little said he never saw a Grace worker himself, but often accommodated doctors who wanted to be present while their patients' X rays were read, explaining to them what he saw and how he drew his conclusions. From those and similar conversations, he understood that the doctors were following up on the sick ones, sending their patients to specialists in Kalispell and Spokane for further tests and treatment—even if they didn't know exactly why the men were getting sick to start with.

One doctor, Woodrow Nelson, conducted spirometer or respiratory function tests on Grace's employees on his own dime, but wrote the company in 1964 and asked for money to take time off and travel to a metropolitan medical center—say, Chicago, in the fall—and analyze these tests. Local doctors, he wrote in the letter, had met to talk about the situation at the mine. "The consensus of local medical opinion was that an important increased incidence of chronic respiratory disease existed in Zonolite employees who had prolonged exposure to dust," he wrote. "Please let me know whether you think Zonolite Division of Grace Company would be interested in pursuing this further. There are many facets to this inhalation problem but this letter is long enough already. Sorry I did not get to see you on your last visit here. My contacts with you and the other members of the company have always been most pleasurable. Sincerely yours, Woodie."

There is no indication that Nelson was ever granted his autumn vacation to the Midwest, but Grace officials did conduct their own lung function tests yearly beginning in 1974. The tests are tricky; it's difficult at times to get an accurate result. While testifying for Les Skramstad in his case against Grace, Spokane doctor Alan Whitehouse related an elaborate set of procedures his office employed to get meaningful results. Grace, however, elected to do these tests internally, entrusting them to Safety Director Harry Eschenbach, manager Earl Lovick, and a few other supervisors with no medical training.

As one of the few games in town, a large employer providing medical insurance to its workers, Grace had a subtle control over the medical community, says Richard Irons, one of the doctors who moved to Libby with Brad Black in 1977. "They basically saw themselves as being in a position where they needed to stay on the good side of the company if they wanted to have their practices thrive," he says. "The company hired and fired people, had insurance. If people didn't have insurance, they wouldn't pay their bills. If people got hurt or sick or in industrial accidents, they had to send people to somebody. Are they going to send them to you or to somebody else? You know, somebody falls and hurts their wrist or something, they've got to be seen. So there was business to come to you if you were friends with the company."

Only scant, circumstantial evidence exists to suggest that any of the doctors, besides Little, knew there was asbestos at the mine, or knew their patients had anything more concrete than abnormal X rays. None of them were pulmonary specialists, and asbestosis was an unusual disease. It's plausible to conclude they thought their patients had nothing more than generic silicosis—miners' lungs—particularly if they weren't looking hard for another explanation. But an incident from 1985 shows that when given the choice, at least one doctor threw his loyalty to the company.

According to a memo written by mine manager Bill McCaig, an investigative reporter from the national consumer watchdog group Public Citizen showed up in town one afternoon in early May 1985 and started asking local doctors about the health of their patients who worked for Grace. "As far as I know, he first contacted Dr. Roger Brus, a Libby surgeon, late yesterday afternoon," McCaig wrote. "Dr. Brus expressed a reluctance to talk to him on the subject since he had no knowledge of who he was or where he was coming from. The man persisted and Dr. Brus told me he played dumb on the subject, so to speak. He gave the man nothing of substance and acted as though asbestos-related disease was something he had read about. ..."

Dr. Black says the nature of the disease made the situation easy to ignore. "I don't think anybody missed anything. I think it was the way it was handled, you know. I've looked back through the workers' records. You'd understand if you understood what the disease is. It moves slow. It's not an easy thing. You look back and say, 'Okay, why didn't you obviously see this going on?' You don't.

"And certainly it's a subtle disease. People don't come in and say, 'I'm short of breath.' What do they do? 'I'm getting older and I just can't do as much as I used to do.' That's a typical story. They're never short of breath really. It's too uncomfortable when they go exert, so they don't do it. They don't understand why they quit mowing their lawn or various things, simple chores you'd think anybody could do. They don't, really. They quit doing it, go do something else, something quieter.

"Yeah, it's real subtle. Most people that have significant disease that we pick up, they're not even aware of it."

And to be honest, he says, the townspeople themselves participated in their own demise by making it impossible to criticize a business that provided paychecks. "It was hard to raise a question of any business operating in Libby that provided jobs, so it was a difficult atmosphere to try to advocate for workers. In one way or another they'd blackball you, and basically that was not an uncommon behavior. Actually the tolerance of varied opinion was just nonexistent."

A lot of men worked felling trees every day—a dangerous job, Black points out—not knowing if they'd come back whole or come back at all. So Libby residents were not the sort of people to tolerate complaints about a little "nuisance dust." In their zeal to work hard and stick together, the town created what was an "incredibly repressive" environment, he says.

Black's partner, Richard Irons, chose to see the best in Libby. As a self-admitted child of the sixties, he interpreted the worst the town had to offer in the best possible light. Irons was no ordinary doctor; he was on a mission to make people's lives better. "I [had] a belief that this could be a community that really took care of its people, was self-sufficient, but not in the old ways, by trying to find some new types of employment for people that wouldn't be boombust," he recalls. "It had to be something besides mining and logging or people weren't going to make it up there."

Fresh out of medical school at Dartmouth, he had volunteered as a missionary doctor in Papau, New Guinea, and Nepal, where he worked in a mountain village hospital under the shadows of Annapurna and Dhaulaghiri. A little self-interest was involved: Irons was a mountain climber, and at the height of his fight against W.R. Grace, this hobby would plunge him to the depths of his soul and help him find the summit again. The story of his time in Libby is a climber's story, and he remembers with bittersweet recall the casualties of those days.

He'd chosen Libby for all kinds of reasons: a friend from medical school, Bruce Hardy, had interned there and recommended it highly. His wife, Karen, was from Missoula, and although she accompanied him abroad, she yearned to return to the mountains of her youth. And he thrived on the satisfaction of giving altruistic medical care; he wanted to go someplace where he was needed and appreciated. Libby had a grand total of five doctors in those days, so it was considered a physician shortage area. Irons, Hardy, and Black made plans to open a clinic in town. "We bought a house and turned it into the Kootenai Clinic," he tells me, punctuating the statement with a harsh, choked-off laugh. How little he knew in what tatters his dreams would lie in a few years.

In addition to the Kootenai Clinic trio, another newcomer, Greg Rice, moved to town and went into private practice that summer. When the four arrived, the medical establishment was less than welcoming.

"They [the other doctors] were formidable in their ability to make a person feel like an outsider," Irons told me in a January 2002 interview. He has moved to Black's old college town of Lawrence, Kansas, but has added far more than simple mileage to his life. He considers Libby, more than fifteen years after he left, through a lens of time and experience. "I suppose the things that stand out from that time the most are resistance to change. The way that they viewed things and the way in which they experienced things was really in the pioneer tradition. You had to live here to really know what was going on. You had to earn your stripes. You're just an outsider until you've been here for quite a while. But with four of us moving in at the same time, that created enough of a stir that the community would never be the same, once these four doctors came in."

Irons plunged into community life. He joined the Rotary Club, directed the choir at the Lutheran Church, and built a house on a bench on the side of a mountain and outfitted it with solar power. He sat on the hospital board, and served for a while as chief of staff and county health officer. Eventually, as he came to treat more and more dying people, he started a hospice program—the first in the region. It was 1978 when he first realized something wasn't quite right with Libby's miners.

"After a year of getting these X rays and pulmonary function tests, I began to ask about them," he says. "Bill McCaig and Earl Lovick invited me to be a consultant and come up and look at Rainy Creek, see what it looked like. I was looking for any extra money I could make, so it seemed like a good thing to do. I went up there and looked at the mine. They told me the stories. Saw the big trucks, saw the dust, saw the people smoking. At that time the management had decided that they would stop smoking and they would try to set an example for the rest of the people that worked there. ... They asked me my opinions on how to look for lung disease in its various forms. That led me to an interest in what was going on there."

By the end of the year, Irons thought he was ready to help Grace deal with its dust problem. The managers at the mine had told him there was tremolite in the dust, but that it was a "short, fat fiber" unlike other forms of asbestos, and therefore less likely to cause disease. He did a little research on his own and concluded that not much good information about tremolite was available. "I also started to look at the fact that more people had lung disease than I ever expected to treat. I looked around and there were a lot of people with great big barrel chests, you know. It looked like emphysema or obstructive lung disease, superficially. And a lot of people that needed oxygen. But then because I was the first internist there, I didn't have anything to compare it to. And no one had been over there really looking for stuff. People who got sick would go either to Kalispell or Missoula or Spokane, so they never had consistent referral patterns."

Then, as his hospice program grew, he noticed a curious thing: "I started going to more funerals. And whenever someone from W.R. Grace would die, there would be Earl Lovick and Bill McCaig. And we waved to each other. We'd be there at the funerals. We'd bury these people, we'd go to their gravesites after the funeral, and watch them put the caskets down and talk to family members." Irons started keeping a list of the dead, a tally of the causes of death. When two cases of mesothelioma showed up, he went to have a talk with Lovick and McCaig.

"I'd say, 'These people died from various forms of lung cancer. And mesothelioma is associated with asbestos, and there are two of these people. Isn't that surprising? That's a very rare tumor.'

"And they said, 'Well, what do you know. We knew about one of these, but gosh, that's pretty unusual, isn't it? But of course if this was asbestos, we'd have a lot more of those. It couldn't be that. And people die from other kinds of lung cancer all the time, you can't really say—and they were smokers, so you can't really say that was the problem.'

"And I said, 'Well, maybe there's a correlation between this and what you're doing up there.'

"'No, no, that's just lung cancer. It's a common cancer.'"

Irons decided to take his concerns to Grace headquarters in Cambridge, Massachusetts, when he had another meeting in nearby Boston. Safety Director Harry Eschenbach agreed to meet with him, and for three hours—including lunch—Irons laid out his plan. He wanted to keep track of employees' physical health, with an emphasis on looking for lung disease, to conduct a retrospective analysis of mortality and illness among present and former Grace employees, and to study Libby's tremolite fiber. Of course, he'd need money from Grace for the project—for his time, for new pulmonary equipment for the hospital. In a letter written after Irons was safely back in Libby, Eschenbach laid out the details of the doctor's proposal. "I expected our discussions to be general and concern ideas he might have to enhance the medical aspects of our safety and health program in Libby. Instead, he had specific proposals which would deeply involve both him and the Libby hospital in the program," Eschenbach wrote. "In summary, I think that Irons sees himself as the Selikoff of the tremolite world and Libby Hospital as the Mt. Sinai of the west."

Very likely, it was the idealistic young Dr. Irons who walked into Eschenbach's office, imagining the great things he could accomplish with Grace's financial backing. But he says he figured out pretty quickly he'd been mistaken, and that Grace wasn't interested in involving outsiders, nor did they want to do any groundbreaking research for the greater good. "For me that was the turning point, because at the meeting, I didn't get a good feeling," he says. "I knew after I'd met him, I'd gotten the bum's rush basically. ... They couldn't wait to get me a plane ticket to get out of town. I mean ... they were cordial but they didn't help me. They denied that any research had been done. They denied that they knew anything. I gave Eschenbach that list of people who had died and he said, 'Oh.' But he didn't do anything."

Grace, of course, had been keeping its own tally. Eschenbach could have told Irons about the X rays taken annually since 1964. He could have shared with Irons the rather ominous results of a 1976 study on tremolite conducted by Dr. William Smith, a researcher at New Jersey's Fairleigh Dickinson University.

Smith, in a 1977 presentation to the Society for Occupational and Environmental Health in Washington, D.C., told the convention that he and his team of researchers had "carried out intrapleural tests in hamsters with three different samples of tremolite." These tremolite samples, he reported, were provided by the Johns-Manville Corporation and the R.T. Vanderbilt Company. Two of the hamster groups contracted varying degrees of fibrosis and tumors from the experiment. What Smith didn't tell the gathering was that he had, in fact, four samples of tremolite to work with. He had asbestos from the Grace's Libby mine.

Smith had previously studied the effects of "platy," or nonfibrous, tremolite talc on mice in 1973, and concluded that this kind of tremolite caused neither cancer nor fibrosis. This, of course, intrigued Grace officials. In 1976 they asked him to take a look at Libby's fibrous tremolite, and the study was funded jointly with Johns-Manville and R.T. Vanderbilt. But Grace's agreement with Smith included a caveat: "All results of our tremolite study will be reported solely to W.R. Grace & Co. and any publication of the findings will be made only by mutual agreement."

Libby's hamsters did not fare so well as the others. One group of rodents was injected with pure tremolite, a second with a 50:50 solution of tremolite and vermiculite. When the scientists had killed ten hamsters from each group ninety days into the experiment, all the Grace animals had fibrosis. On a scale of 0 to 4, with 4 considered "extensive" fibrosis, the average was 3.3 and 3.6 respectively. Additionally, by the end of the experiment, there were five mesotheliomas from each Libby group, out of only twenty-two total surviving hamsters. The control group, by contrast, showed no fibrosis, no mesothelioma, and only one unrelated cancer.

These results were never published, not revealed to any government agency until decades later, and certainly not confided by Harry Eschenbach to Dr. Richard Irons.

A few months later, Irons turned up the heat. He followed up his visit to Grace's headquarters with a letter to Eschenbach, stating his intent to proceed with a study even if Grace declined to be involved. "If conclusions are reached on the basis of this that suggest that the public be made aware of these health hazards," he wrote, "I would at that point feel justified and required to make this information public." Grace's reaction was immediate. Eschenbach wrote Libby manager Bob Oliverio and Grace executive Jack Wolter to warn them. He saw Irons's demands as blackmail. "As you can conclude from his memo, Irons is 'turning the screw.' He is apparently looking for financial support from Grace to do a study of Libby Zonolite employees. I think that his latest letter more or less puts his position on the line. We either play the game his way or he is going to blow the whistle. I have not decided what the best response to this thrust is at this time."

Attempts to contact Eschenbach, a former special agent with the U.S. Army Counterintelligence Corps who now lives in Massachusetts, were unsuccessful.

Irons, however, did not have enough information to go public. All he had were some sick miners and his suspicions. He told his patients who were Grace employees what he thought was happening to them; he told their wives to take precautions when washing their husbands' dusty clothes. He kept his list and in his capacity as county health officer, told the county commissioners he was keeping such a record. Their response was cautious: "'We've got to look out for the overall economic interests of the community,'" he says they told him. "'Unless we have some proof of this, there's nothing else we could do.'" He tried to get the medical records of the rest of Libby's miners, but was stalled at every turn—other doctors guarded their patients' records jealously. While the hospital's records—with Dr. Little's X rays—were open to Grace officials, Irons says they were closed to him. Meanwhile, Irons's practice suffered. Grace's managers stopped coming to him for their health care. Eschenbach sent him a letter meant to reassure him that Grace had everything under control. Then one weekend, Irons's own life spun completely out of control.

"I had continued to be involved with the Sierra Club. I hung out with Forest Service folks, climbed mountains and fished, camped, enjoyed the area. I mean, that's why I went there.

"One time when I was climbing Snowshoe Peak, which is not too far—Snowshoe Peak is part of the Cabinets, and it's the second-highest peak in that area. On the way down from that, we were crossing a narrow ice field and I was the first person in line. I wasn't paying much attention. We'd climbed the peak, and I'd climbed a lot of other stuff. We were just coming down, but I slipped and fell down this ice field 125 feet when one of the steps came loose. I came up against a rock wall and my arms were up like that," he says, holding his arms above his head. "And I was cut right here.

It knocked all the muscle off my arm, had a huge gash in my arm to the point where I could look down and see my arm bone." Irons rolls up his shirt sleeve to show me the scar high on the inside of his upper left arm. "So I was with Black and one of the dentists. They gave me a few pain pills and I had to walk out or stay there until the next day and wait for a helicopter to get me out. By then I thought I'd have osteomyelitis, infection of the bone. So I walked out. I was lucky. I was spared. I could have broken my neck. I could have died."

What he did, in the process of a long recovery and painful physical therapy, was become addicted to pain pills. "Some of the doctors in town were alcoholic. No one cared about that. But if you were addicted to pain pills, then you were a drug addict," he says, a tone of resentment still in his voice after nearly two decades. "That was a different thing."

His marriage began to crumble. His wife, Karen, became a fundamentalist Christian, striking out on a spiritual path that clashed with Irons's own more tolerant Buddhist leanings. She had a brain tumor from which she died in 1992, but in the early 1980s, her condition was as yet undiagnosed, and neither Karen nor Richard understood the forces that were controlling them. A breakthrough came, a lifeline for the doctor, when in 1983 he was asked to join an expedition to climb Mt. Everest from the Tibetan east side. He eagerly accepted, a chance to fulfill a long-held dream of visiting Tibet and climbing one of the world's most formidable mountains. Of course, he had to get clean to do it. "That was part of what convinced me I really wasn't a drug addict. I was strong. I didn't use while I was doing that, of course. That would have been foolish. I could give up drugs; I was strong. I could go on another mission."

When he returned from the expedition, Irons entered treatment, then came back to Libby in 1985. "I had to make a decision about what to do with my life. I'd been there eight years. Was I going to stay there? I had some support for staying. Life was difficult enough. I had a wife, two kids. We had our problems; my wife had her problems." Meanwhile, another internist had moved to town and had been helping Irons with his practice. "He really preferred to work alone. Once I was gone, he just wanted to carry on what at that time was a declining practice. He wanted to buy me out, so I sold out to him." Although his wife decided she wanted to stay in Libby, Irons moved to the state's capital in Helena, a three-hour drive from Libby just east of the Continental Divide. He dropped his campaign to fix Grace's problems and focused on his own. Even in retrospect, he tells me, there's not much more he could have done.

In his new life, Irons runs an addiction treatment center for professionals. While you can still see the compact climber's body under a moderate layer of middle-age girth, Irons says he has let that part of his life go, too. He works in an upscale office park at the edge of the Lawrence city limits. The nearby rolling hills have a subtle grace despite the overlay of agriculture. And while Irons does not seem to be the kind of man who will wallow in regret, his voice carries a hint of wistfulness over the loss of the northern Rockies' spectacular beauty as a daily presence in his life. Although there are more than a few people in Libby who will tell you Grace pressured him to leave town, Irons refuses to lay blame at the corporation's doorstep. "I pretty much figure that's my own stuff. I decided to leave town. They certainly weren't sorry to see me leave."

Richard Irons was a fortunate man; he was given the chance to make amends of sorts for leaving Libby when Grace's victims began suing the corporation. They tracked him down and he agreed to testify in court, to advocate for Libby's sick and dying. His life had come full-circle when two months after our talk, Richard Irons died in the home he shared with his wife, Kirsten, of cardiac arrhythmia. He was fifty-three years old.

MORE THAN ONE HUNDRED YEARS after asbestosis made its first appearance in the medical literature, Dr. Alan Whitehouse finds himself answering "I don't know" to most questions I ask about the progression of the disease. This is significant: Whitehouse works in Spokane, Washington, and so is the doctor of choice for many Libby residents. He reckons he is probably treating a larger number of patients with asbestos-related diseases than is any other doctor in the United States. This "treatment," however, is an unsatisfactory business.

"Well, there's some things you can treat," he says. "You can treat fluid in the chest, which occurs in a fair number of these people. You can look for and treat lung cancers and potentially cure them. A lot of these people develop asthma which you can treat," he says. "But as far as the underlying process, it's not treatable at this point. And so it's been a progressive thing for most people, but not always. It's not clear what are the factors that make it progressive and what are the factors that don't make it progressive, why some person remains exactly the same for ten years and why another person goes downhill. That's not clear." Whitehouse estimates that the fibrosis in about a third of his asbestos patients is not advancing—at least not that he can tell. Whether it will, he has no idea.

Whitehouse was an expert witness for Les Skramstad when he took W.R. Grace to court, and in that case he took Skramstad's jury, step-by-step, on a tour of asbestos-sick lungs. The biology is not too complicated: the trachea, the windpipe, is connected to a pair of bronchial air tubes, which, as they descend into each lung, divide further into branches that wind through our upper and lower lung lobes, ending in bunches of air sacs that resemble grapes. In these sacs, the alveoli, our lungs exchange oxygen for carbon dioxide. The structure holding all this in place is the interstitium. The lungs are covered, like the rest of our organs, with protective mesothelial cells. In the case of the lungs, there are actually two layers of mesothelial cells called the pleura—thin as Saran Wrap and very fragile, Whitehouse says. The space in between is filled with lubricating fluid that protects the lungs as they expand and contract.

Asbestos fibers can affect every part of this system. The fibers are heavier than air and so begin by settling into the lungs' lower lobes. Then the scarring begins, an endless cycle of irritation, inflammation, and calcification. The fibers may work their way into the pleural linings, the resulting scars slowly growing into a crenulated straightjacket that prevents the lungs from expanding. A doctor with a stethoscope can hear this development: a sound like crinkling cellophane called rales. If the pleura tears, the protective fluid leaks into the chest cavity, a phenomenon referred to as pleural effusions. "The lung is sort of like a bellows," Whitehouse explains. "The only reason it inflates is because ... when you take a deep breath, there's a vacuum. If you put a hole in this lining, all the air will escape and the lung will collapse ... it'll push the lung down and the lung can fill or the space can fill with fluids."

The asbestos fibers also may infiltrate the interstitum, encircling the air sacs and cutting off the exchange of gases. The upper lobes may overcompensate, the patient developing asthma or emphysema. At this point a patient may have trouble exhaling as well as inhaling, as air gets trapped in the lungs. All this puts extra strain on the heart. The patient feels as if he were suffocating. Eventually he will.

Some patients—mainly smokers—develop lung cancer (though at a rate three times higher than smokers with no asbestos exposure, and ninety-two times higher than nonsmokers with no asbestos exposure). Sometimes the mesothelial cells go wild. Although there is ongoing research into whether there is a viral component in some cases of mesothelioma, the disease is such a rare cancer that the federal government has no statistics on its occurrence in the general population. It is associated almost exclusively with asbestos exposure.

Whitehouse ticks off the factors involved in Les Skramstad's diagnosis: "First off ... he had a history of asbestos exposure for approximately two years plus or minus a bit in a dusty atmosphere that is known to have high quantities of asbestos fibers. Second, on exam he had a restrictive chest and he had rales. On history he had significant shortness of breath and difficulty with his breathing, and then he has the chest X-ray findings of the calcification of his diaphragm, the interstitial changes in his lungs on both sides, the pleural thickening, which are all hallmarks of asbestosis."

The fact that Les hadn't been exposed to asbestos for nearly forty years makes no difference, Whitehouse says, because the disease is a cumulative one. "That means whatever you inhale today is there forever. ..."

With 450 patients sick from Libby's vermiculite mine, added to his regular pulmonary and internal medicine practice, Whitehouse has had little time for the journalists who are interested in Libby's notoriety. Getting him to sit down with me took a few months, and he's worked with very few of the reporters who have come calling. It seems that for him, every day is busy, every week is a long one. He makes it clear that I had better move things right along. Though I've read his testimony on asbestosis, my questions are a little too pedestrian, and he answers me laconically until we hit upon the topic of the fix people are finding themselves in. "A lot of them have Medicare, but Medicare's a problem and they can't afford the supplemental insurance. People up there aren't very wealthy, there's a lot of drug costs, so I don't know what will happen," he says, shaking his head. "I really don't."

Whitehouse tag-teams with Dr. Brad Black. A fast driver, according to his secretaries, Whitehouse makes the four-hour trip to Libby in three hours every month or so to meet with Black, look over X rays, and collaborate on treatment. Whitehouse's involvement is essential—there is still no lung specialist in Libby. Nor, he says, is there likely to ever be, given the community's constantly struggling economy.

Black is more optimistic, though even he says Grace can't be counted on to continue its financial support of his clinic indefinitely. "Unless there's some financial gain from them doing it, it's not an integrity thing, that's for sure," he says. When Grace's funding dries up (which is likely once the company's finances are litigated), Black is hoping for a government-inspired White Lung program to take up the burden—Libby is, after all, looking at new cases being diagnosed for potentially the next forty years.

ANDRIJ HOLIAN MAY HOLD the key to answering some of the medical questions Drs. Whitehouse and Black are struggling with. If his work proves productive, scientists will know a lot more about the reasons why asbestos fibers cause disease, and in turn will be able to provide doctors with effective tools for treatment—something beyond the pills and inhalers that now just ease patients toward death.

Holian is reluctant to say that fate brought him to the cutting edge of asbestos research in the United States, but he admits the coincidences are curious. A quarter of a century after he fell in love with the mountains as an undergraduate summer researcher at Montana State University in Bozeman, Holian finds himself in charge of the Center for Environmental Health Sciences from a cramped office on the state's other major campus, at the University of Montana, about four hours south of Libby in Missoula. Holian is an Ohio native, raised just outside Toledo in the heart of the Rust Belt. And like all good midwestern boys, he chose his college—Bowling Green State University—primarily for its forty-five-minute proximity to hometown and family. By the end of his sophomore year, however, he had been struck with a mild case of wanderlust, and started looking into undergraduate research programs. "I applied to ones at Case Western in Ohio and to a bunch of other schools, and Montana State was the one that was furthest away. I'd never really been away from the Chicago-Cleveland belt where my family lived. I decided that I needed to really see another part of the United States.

"So I went to Bozeman and my first four hours of being there was standing outside the doorway looking up at the mountains there. I'd never really seen that before. It was just amazing to me."

Holian loved everything about that summer in the mountains, so he came back to Bozeman to get his Ph.D. in chemistry in 1975 before reluctantly admitting that he couldn't stay. "I was disappointed in the fact that I had to leave, but Montana offers very few employment opportunities," he says, "especially for people with higher degrees."

He moved around a bit, first to the University of Pennsylvania where he rubbed elbows with scientists working on silica and lung problems, then to Villanova University in Pennsylvania, before finally settling down in Houston. There, where the green hills of Texas meet the Gulf Coast of Mexico, Holian joined the faculty of the University of Texas's Health Science Center and stayed for sixteen years—until circumstances began converging in his life, drawing him back to the mountains.

"A student in the school of public health had found out that I was the only person on the whole Texas medical center campus, in fact, that was doing work with what could be construed as lung diseases, environmental lung diseases. And so he said that they're going to throw him out of the school of public health and he wants to get his doctorate, unless he can find a mentor who will work with him on a project."

It was a long shot. Holian's research dealt with the factors that activate the immune cells in people's lungs, but his experience with specific lung diseases was limited to what he had gained through osmosis in the Pennsylvania lab. Nevertheless, he agreed to be a mentor, thinking, "Maybe we can do some work with asbestos fibers. And so in fact that's how it really started, from a desperate student that came to my laboratory."

Eventually the wanderlust struck again. After a decade and a half in Texas, Holian had had enough of the state, and more than enough of the summers. He began thinking of another move. "I'd always kind of wanted to come back to Montana, but there had to be a situation to come back. A colleague of mine asked me to look at a job at Yale, it was the director of an institute there. I put him off, put him off for six months, then later on I ... got tired of it and said, 'Okay, I'll look, but I need to look at someplace else, at least one other place.' So I opened up a magazine that has job positions for professions in science. I looked at that, I was browsing through it, and I ran across an advertisement that they were looking for a director for a new center here [in Missoula]. So I said, 'Wow.'"

About the same time, Holian won a grant from the National Institutes of Health to look at silica- and asbestos-related lung diseases. At that point, both he and the NIH officials imagined he would focus on silica. "It's something that was still more of a real-time problem than asbestos. Asbestos-related diseases seemed to be something that was really not happening that much anymore. So that was more or less the status of affairs.

"And about the time I was looking to move up here, and I was interviewing, was when the news really started breaking out about the Libby situation. And so I've shifted the emphasis more to the asbestos side of the project. Great coincidence, it might be called. There's in fact not that many people, investigators, working on asbestos-related diseases because it wasn't considered to be terribly relevant anymore. In fact, a year ago when I was talking to the National Institute of Health folks, they were telling me, 'Try to couch this in broader terms.' And now they're not emphasizing that as much anymore because they're appreciating the significance of the Libby situation."

The significance of Libby lies in the potential scope of the problem. Even Holian, who speaks with the careful caveats of a scientist, agrees that the possible health consequences are both considerable and continuing. "Even though the exposures were obviously greatest for those people working in the mines up there and the processing plants, if you have sensitive individuals around the country who have been working with the vermiculite up there, whether it's Toledo, Ohio, or Kalamazoo, Michigan, or wherever, if they were handling fairly large amounts of it in gardening or insulation, and they were susceptible individuals, it may be a greater problem." And because there was such a great effort to get rid of commercial asbestos products in the 1980s, health care professionals have generally assumed that asbestos is an isolated problem from the past. "So this may also be happening around the country," Holian says. "There have been possibly misdiagnoses all around the country where this stuff may have been shipped, or other places in the world even. Because it wasn't supposed to be around, therefore it can't be this, it must be something else.

"If everybody had the opportunity of looking back now, we may find that there is much more asbestos-related disease all around than what we think, because it's not supposed to have been there, therefore it had been excluded.

"Nobody was looking for it."

With Libby, everything has changed. Doctors and state and federal health agencies are finally beginning to consider asbestos-related diseases. Holian's job is to outfit them with the tools for treating it.

Fibrosis, he tells me, is a form of chronic lung inflammation, a broad category of diseases that includes asthma. Fibrosis can be caused by cotton dust, coal dust, asbestos, or silica exposure. "And then here's this broad category called idiopathic pulmonary fibrosis for which they don't know the cause of it," Holian says. "There are no effective treatments for any of these kinds of lung fibrosis, and it has nothing to do with asbestos specifically. The fact is, this is not well understood." By getting a handle on what Holian calls the "mechanism" of fibrosis—determining how the disease takes place—the University of Montana researchers could be finding the key to treatment for a whole range of sick people.

Holian's team of scientists is attacking the asbestos problem on four fronts. First, they are looking for genetic markers among Libby residents that either predispose people to develop asbestos-related disease or protect them from doing so. "We can do that by comparing individuals that have been similarly exposed up in Libby, and looking at their DNA makeup and finding out what's different about the people who have the exposure, and who have and do not have the disease," he says. "The ideal would be if we can identify genes that are conferring protection. That gives us tremendous hope that we'll be able then to develop a therapeutic approach." In a related second study the researchers are looking for specific genes that encourage tumor development in response to asbestos exposure. To that end the doctors are paying Libby residents $100 to undergo a rather uncomfortable procedure called lavage. "They stick an open tube down into your lungs, put some fluid in there, and then bring it back out," Holian explains. "That's the only way of getting the cells from the lung that we're particularly interested in there." (Even as she encourages her friends and neighbors to participate in Holian's projects, Gayla Benefield jokes about this genetic research: "They're going to find out we're all related up here.")

A third tack is related to Holian's specialty: the immune system. He has noticed a high incidence of autoimmune disease (another broad category of illnesses, these affecting the immune system, encompassing everything from leukemia to AIDS) among Libby residents and is curious if there is a connection to the high rates of asbestos exposure. One of his researchers is working on a formal study to quantify Holian's hunch by comparing the incidence of autoimmune diseases among Libby residents with that in a similar population in Missoula (both groups with a northern European background) and then with the incidence in the general U.S. population. Fourth, Holian himself is working with the asbestos fiber specific to Libby. He explains that the mechanism of fibrosis may boil down to the fibers' effects on the lungs' immune system. "If you have shifting immune status in the small airways, then you're precipitating, exacerbating asthma. It's the one thing we're looking at with some particles: if you're doing that in the lung parenchyma, then you're precipitating diseases such as lung fibrosis." He is testing his hypothesis—in simple terms, that asbestos is altering the immune environment of the lung—in part by comparing Libby's tremolite with other kinds of asbestos. "Principally, the asbestos fibers fall into two broad categories: serpentine asbestos, which is the chrysotile asbestos, also called sometimes 'white asbestos.' This is the most heavily used form. That accounts for probably about 90 percent of all the asbestos that has been mined and utilized."

Libby's tremolite falls into the second category, a noncommercial form called amphibole asbestos that's not so well characterized. "That's a very broad class of asbestos fibers. They are not flexible; they're straight shards. They all have the same backbone, but they're varied upon the associated ions that give it certain characteristics, color in some cases. Crocidolite is sometimes called "blue asbestos," has a fair amount of iron associated with it, for example. And then the asbestos that's up in Libby has varying amounts of sodium and manganese and some other ions associated with it.

"Amphibole fibers survive in the lung longer than serpentine fibers. That is why they are considered more harmful."

Specifically, Holian is interested in how the different kinds of asbestos affect the immune status of the lungs, first in terms of the "relative potency" wielded by each asbestiform, and second, "the difficulty in being eliminated. If you clear a particle out, then presumably whatever effect is being caused is more likely to be transient. If you can't remove a particle, then it's more likely to be chronic. ... But if it's a matter of controlling the immune status of the lung, then hopefully we can suppress at least that type of activity."

Medical opinion moves slowly, and Holian realizes that he's not only tackling mysteries of lung biology but also the common medical sense that asbestos-related diseases are so obsolete—or limited to people who were employed at known hot spots, such as shipyard workers or those in the construction trade before modern asbestos standards were put in place—as to deter study. But with the EPA estimating that at least 15 million buildings in the U.S. contain Libby's vermiculite (other estimates go as high as 35 million buildings), there's ample reason to pay closer attention to asbestos diseases. "There are what's called conventional wisdom out there, and when you're trying to change conventional wisdom, it takes a while to convince other people that, you know, let's throw this idea away, or at least accept that there might be something else here going on. And in part that's what we've tried to do over the past few years. This whole situation here has really been an interesting meld of a need and what we've already b en working on in this direction."

Kinship

Carrie and Bob Dedrick were not chosen at random to host Governor Marc Racicot for his photo-op visit to a home with Zonolite insulation in late 1999, on his first trip to Libby since the news broke about the asbestos problems here. As the press, the EPA, and politicians crowd into the Dedricks' modest home on Colorado Avenue, a few blocks west of downtown Libby and south of the river, Carrie lets the governor know this: "We're related, you know." It seems the two have a great-great-grandfather in common. Racicot was not aware of this, and the two talk and soon discover that they get Christmas cards from at least one shared relative.

But the Dedricks don't waste much time swapping stories with the governor. It's their chance to make one political point, and they

take it. Montana's Republican senator Conrad Burns is cosponsor-
ing a bill called the Fairness in Asbestos Compensation Act. The
measure is being pushed by asbestos companies in the name of efficiency, but it would in effect keep Libby victims out of court.
"There's been a bill they're trying to get in that [Montana Representative Rick] Hill and Burns are supporting, and it's going to be
very detrimental to the people who live here," Bob Dedrick explains to the governor. "The problem in Libby is not associated with
the rest of the asbestos problem. They're not even related. In Libby
we're doing a good job taking care of these things in the court."

The governor tells Bob he hasn't had a chance to look at the bill
yet, but promises to do so. Then Bob gets to his biggest personal
concern: his grandkids. He and Carrie have seven of them, including two of Jenan Swenson's daughters. One set of parents is reluctant to let the kids stay with the Dedricks until they know whether
the home is safe. "We wanted to know because of our grandkids
and great-grandkids. We have it [asbestosis], but we're afraid to
have the children here until we know."

Racicot reassures the Dedricks that the state, despite its past
neglect in Libby, will be vigilant making sure that people's homes
are safe. As the other reporters crowd into the Dedricks' kitchen
to hear what else the governor will say, I stay in the living room
and catch the attention of Mark Simonich, a former logging executive who ran the state's Department of Environmental Quality in
the 1990s. Simonich also has a history in Libby—he lived here for
a couple of years during his mid-twenties. One very cold winter, he
says, he added Zonolite insulation to the home he was living in.

He is reluctant to talk about the mistakes his predecessors
made, and wants to focus on current health risks. "But," I persist,
"don't you need to fix whatever procedures were broken?"

"From our perspective, if we were permitting a vermiculite mine
today, we'd look at it very differently," he says. "From the stand-
point of occupational safety, the laws that were put on the books
in the '70s deal much better with occupational exposure."

But, I press further, a lot of people were exposed up here in the
'70s, despite the laws.

He seems exasperated with the question. "People might be as willing to do what they did with it. It wasn't that you knew you were exposed and there was a quick onset of sickness. It really takes many, many, many years, decades. So unless people see something physical happen, they don't always accept that it's hazardous." It's a rationalization for gross negligence, and I suspect we both know it. It's difficult for a bureaucrat to admit to the enormity of the mistakes made here, and Simonich does not stick his neck out to do so.

The governor's aides are anxious to move along. A public meeting is scheduled for later tonight, and the EPA has more stops for Racicot to make this evening. We all thank the Dedricks, and they wish us good-bye. We leave them standing alone, silhouetted against the dim light of their kitchen, stand-ins for all the grandparents not lucky enough to be related to the governor.

SIX

The Watchdogs Take a Nap

MARC RACICOT IS ON HIS home turf in Libby's Memorial Gymnasium. The fifty-three-year-old governor grew up in this town where he is remembered as a basketball star, the coach's son who led his team to its first and only state championship in 1966. His family's roots were planted in the Montana Territory in the 1860s; his grandfather struck out for Libby in 1917, where he worked as a logging camp cook for the J. Neils Lumber Company. Racicot's wholesome background is part of a well-crafted image that made him the state's most powerful political figure of the 1990s and brought him to the attention of presidential candidate George W. Bush and ultimately to a position at the head of the Republican National Committee. But one night just before Christmas 1999, the thin, hatchet-faced Republican politician returned to the old gym to face a less-than-friendly hometown crowd, more than 200 former neighbors looking for answers about the sickness that had hit their community like a slam-dunk from out of nowhere.

Racicot had a lot to answer for. As a Libby native, he must have known something of the miners' plight. And as a state office-holder—first winning the attorney general's seat in 1988, then serving two terms as governor—the star ballplayer missed his chance to be a champion for his people. Racicot knew there were lawsuits, knew there was controversy over returning Grace's reclamation bond, but despite all his years in Libby—his small-town biography used to great political advantage—the governor maintains he had no idea there was anything amiss with the mine. At least that's what he has told the journalists who ask him. I am incredulous and put the question to him a little differently: Did he personally know anyone who was sick? Who had died? "I didn't know until the most recent reports," he says, pausing as if the question summoned faces and memories. "Some people I knew from when I grew up here, I know from media reports, have suffered and died. I haven't spoken with the family members."

Then he slips back into politician mode. "I do know it's a matter of grave and serious concern. It's particularly piercing and searing to know people who've had these challenges visited upon them."

Racicot's concern for his hometown rings hollow to many of the victims here, but the man himself can hardly be blamed, single-handedly, for the circumstances that have brought us all to the gym tonight. Because Montana was built on mining, and the industry's agenda dictated events under the copper-domed capitol in Helena nearly to the end of the twentieth century. Beginning in the late 1800s, Montana's blood ran gold, silver, and copper through veins that fed the bank accounts of East Coast capitalists. The mightiest of these were the copper barons, Marcus Daly and William Clark, prospectors who began by working other men's claims but built rival mining empires and fought each other vicariously using the state's unions, politicians, and voters as their pawns. Eventually, Daly's Anaconda Company emerged as the victor. As historian Michael Malone put it, "the massive copper deposits of Butte brought some of the world's greatest capitalists onto the Montana scene, and they, in turn, brought development and a measure of prosperity. ... Unfortunately, the Treasure State also had to pay a high price, for copper came to dominate its economy and to rule the roost politically, sometimes with grim results."

Clark and Daly bought their power—the two regularly bribed legislators, and Clark was accused in 1899 of buying the grand jurors charged with investigating the accusations of bribery (the reported cost: $10,000 apiece). But by the time the Anaconda Company hit its apex after Daly's death, the company owned the state. In 1915 the Anaconda Copper Mining Company had the budget of a small country and treated Montana as a colony: "With assets of $118 million and a copper production capacity of 300 million pounds a year, the Company was the giant of the world's copper industry," Malone wrote. "To many observers, both inside and outside the state, Montana appeared to be the classic example of a 'one-company state,' a commonwealth where one corporation ruled."

Even if Anaconda had declined to exert direct influence in Helena, the company probably would have dominated Montana's economic and political life by sheer mass. Anaconda owned most of the state's newspapers, many of the motels and stores. The company held title to more than a half million acres of timberland and ran free bars for legislators. And it had what Malone calls a "Siamese Twin" in the form of the Montana Power Company, the state's electric utility, which was owned by Anaconda president John D. Ryan until 1928. From the start the state's mining industry was singled out for special treatment. Montana's original constitution, ratified in 1889, spelled out a liberal policy under which mining companies' taxes were assessed solely on their net proceeds. In his 1919 book, *The Taxation of Mines in Montana*, Missoula professor Louis Levine reported that the state's mining companies generate almost half of Montana's gross domestic product, but account for only 8 percent of the state's tax revenue. Although Levine called for the reform of the system with language almost mathematical in its objectivity, his conclusion that mining should be treated like any other business was inescapably radical and he was soon fired.

"The Company applied the same heavy hand to its workers. If a union threatened to strike, the Company would close the mine until the workers surrendered," wrote journalist Heather Abel in a 1997 report on the rise and fall of Montana's mining industry. "It used Pinkerton detectives and spies to divide the unions. This last strategy worked so well that in 1914, union factions rioted against each other at Butte's Miners' Union Hall, reducing it to rubble."

Reforms came gradually as the mighty Anaconda relaxed its grip on the state, beginning about mid-century. As it diversified and expanded in other countries (most notably South America), Anaconda lost interest in Montana. The company sold its newspaper empire in 1959 to Iowa's Lee Enterprises, and unloaded its nearly defunct copper mines on the Atlantic Richfield Company (ARCO) in 1977. The resulting Berkeley Pit is now a tourist attraction in itself, as the largest man-made hole in the world. (The Pit also serves as the headwaters of the largest Superfund site in the United States, a 100-mile-long river of heavy metals that comes to rest against the Milltown Dam just outside Missoula.)

The tide of public sentiment that would eventually dilute the industry's influence began turning in 1972, when Montana adopted a new constitution that announced the state's citizens had the right to live in "a clean and healthful environment." While mining companies insisted the provision was simply a rhetorical ideal to which they might aspire, the state supreme court declared in 1999 that the right was a fundamental one on which Montanans could count to protect their air and water. The constitution was followed in the 1970s by a series of laws regulating hard-rock mining, protecting water quality, and requiring reclamation of mine sites. In 1975, lawmakers passed a 33 percent coal severance tax, the highest in the nation.

It was one of the most far-reaching pieces of legislation from that decade, says Attorney General Mike McGrath who, as an assistant in the office he now leads, helped defend the constitutionality of the law when it was appealed to the state supreme court. "That was enacted specifically to offset the sort of boom-and-bust cycle," McGrath explains. "Again, you've got a colonial economy. They come in, the commodity price is good, so they mine, then they go out of business; they go bankrupt, you know. They're gone and we get stuck with the social costs, the environmental costs. The coal tax, the idea was, we're going to tax these guys 33 percent and they're going to pay some of the costs for increased schools, roads, police and fire protection, the kind of government services that they benefit from. We're going to make them pay that up front, but in addition we're going to sock a bunch of this money away for the very purposes that we've been talking about so that the future generations don't get left holding the bag. That was a far-reaching decision."

Anaconda put up its last fight when the 1975 legislature ordered a review—and subsequent overhaul—of the state's mine tax policy.

According to a 1978 report issued by the Revenue Oversight Committee, the net proceeds tax allowed Anaconda and others to
claim so many deductions that there was rarely much profit left for
the state to tax. "During the past 50 years, the net proceeds of
metal mines ... has always comprised less than five percent of the
total tax base of the state and often less than one percent," wrote
the report's author, Teresa Olcott Cohea. Although the legislature
changed the law regarding metal mines to close many of these
loopholes (a move that Anaconda unsuccessfully took to the
state's Tax Appeals Board), as a nonmetal mine Libby was exempt
and still taxed on its largely imagined "net proceeds." According
to Cohea's numbers, the vermiculite industry (of which Grace was
the only substantial member) from 1972 to 1976 claimed only
.0046 percent of its gross proceeds as taxable income. The mine
managers, according to one local politician, fought to reduce that
tax burden even further.

Paula Darko, a home economics teacher who served in the legislature in the early 1980s, recalls being bullied to support a measure
allowing even more deductions for the company.

"Earl Lovick and Bill McCaig, who was the manager up there,
they came to the legislature and said, 'Paula, this bill helps us with
our taxes. We're taxed on net proceeds and some of the exemptions
we want to have aren't legal, so we want to change the law so that
we can get some more deductions allowed on our net proceeds. ...'

"And I said, 'Well, that sounds reasonable,' so then I went
ahead and signed on the bill. ... And they're over there wining and
dining me, and I got to thinking, 'You know, if we lower their
taxes, it means a loss to schools, it means a loss to our tax base.'
And it was substantial; it was a lot of money."

Darko withdrew her support and the measure failed. "I got up on
the floor of the House and said, 'I can't support this bill. I'm taking
my name off this bill. Our schools will lose money, and who is able
to pay this tax bill? W.R. Grace or the people of my community?'
And the bill died. [McCaig] called me out in the hall and he called
me every name. He was so angry, he could hardly speak. So then I
became Dumb Darko. And his vendetta was to get me defeated in

the next election. I mean, he did everything he could. My name at the Chamber of Commerce was Dumb Darko." Stung by McCaig's spite, Darko says she was happy to have served only one term. "People in this town, I don't know. They're just mean. ... I've spent too much of my life and too much of my good health trying to help people who didn't appreciate it. Call you up in the middle of the night and tell you off. I got defeated in the election the last time I ran, and I think the Lord was looking out for me because I don't know that I could have done it anymore. It was just getting to be too nasty." She intends to leave Libby as soon as she retires and move back to her hometown of Great Falls along the big open of the Rocky Mountain Front.

In Anaconda's absence, the state's political scene dissolved into a cacophony of interests: logging companies and sawmill workers, conservationists and ranchers, anglers and real estate developers, unions and relocated tourists. Movie stars. Big-game hunters. In Helena a consortium of mining companies organized loosely under the auspices of the Montana Mining Association still wielded substantial influence through the 1990s. These companies could send a lobbyist into the capitol with the text of a bill saved on a computer disk, hand it to a legislator, and expect it to become law. Governor Racicot signed two such measures in 1995, weakening the state's water quality laws. But between the shifting economy and the gaining momentum of conservation ideals, the mining industry began to lose ground.

In 1997, Racicot's top environmental official, Department of Environmental Quality chief Mark Simonich, was accused by his own spokesperson of "spin-doctoring and truth twisting" in an apparent attempt to make things easier on the industries he was supposed to be regulating. Cathy Siegner, a fiery redhead who chooses her words carefully, resigned in an embarrassingly public way, saying that Simonich and his deputy, Curt Chisholm, seemed to be answering first to the business community and only second to the law and citizens of Montana. "Conditions in the department have made it increasingly difficult, if not impossible, to effectively do my job of trying to enhance the level of trust and confidence the public and press hold in its activities," Siegner wrote in her resignation letter. "I refer to the appalling degree of spin-doctoring and truth-twisting being performed by you and Curt Chisholm on department issues in the press.

"I will not stand by on the state payroll and watch you stretch the truth in order to further some agenda that is neither publicly discussed nor collectively supported." The governor dismissed Siegner's accusations after conducting his own investigation of the matter, but the allegations came at an interesting time for the mining industry. A Colorado-based company, Canyon Resources, was in the final stages of applying for a permit to mine gold at the headwaters of the Big Blackfoot, the beloved river of Norman Maclean's novella, *A River Runs Through It*. As the river's advocates were gearing up for what they expected to be an ugly and probably physical confrontation, Montana environmentalists capitalized on that groundswell by turning to the ballot box. In the last half of the 1990s, voters would approve a ban on cyanide-heap leach mining, the preferred method of corporate gold-diggers (smaller operations tended to use the old-fashioned placer method of mining for gold), and would reject a bid to tighten water quality regulations in a campaign where out-of-state mining companies outspent environmentalists six to one. (This last measure failed in the same election cycle in which voters passed restrictions on corporate campaign financing; Missoula political columnist Bill Chaloupka characterized the schizophrenic results as the electorate saying, "Stop me before I vote again.")

In the wake of King Copper's abdication, its heirs—gold and silver—found themselves rebuffed in attempts to excavate near national treasures. Plagued by low gold prices and the ban on cyanide mining, Canyon Resources shelved its plan to mine the Blackfoot. Also in 1998, Canadian mining giant Noranda was forced to give up its bid to extract gold from the area between Yellowstone National Park and the Absaroka-Beartooth Wilderness. While the state has approved plans for the Mexico-based ASARCO to dig 100 million tons of copper and silver out from under the Cabinet-Yaak Wilderness area in Libby's corner of the state, the mining

giant faces a tough battle from conservationists who have a powerful ally in the form of the Wilderness Act on their side.

Approximately 6,500 Montanans are employed in the mining
industry—1.1 percent of the total workforce. The industry con-
tributes about 3 percent to the state's annual gross production and
pays about 6 percent of the state's taxes. Citing a lack of funds, the
Montana Mining Association closed its doors in 2001. Like the
Chicago Bulls without Jordan or the Libby Loggers without Racicot,
the absence of Anaconda had converted the industry into just another special interest.

LIBBY WAS FAR REMOVED both geographically and politically
from those early battles that turned Butte into a combat zone. The
town and its industries were of one mind. They were, so far as the
citizens were concerned, all on the same team. There weren't even
any strikes in Libby during labor's heyday in the rest of the state.
But both Zonolite and the Grace corporation benefited from King
Copper's reign. State laws favored the company, and in the case of
Libby it meant that Grace could use the non-retroactive 1959
Occupational Disease Act as a shield against responsibility for
those first sick workers by claiming they'd been made ill prior to
the passage of the law. State inspectors wielded little power; even
as Ben Wake spoke in terms of "maximum allowable concentrations," he lamented that he could do little more than complain
about the dust in Libby. In a 1964 letter to the union, Wake wrote,
"enforcement provisions of the Industrial Hygiene Act of 1939 are
very poor. The [attorney general's] office has not strengthened the
Act and we can only use certain portions of the Act to achieve
compliance with recommendations." And Wake's reports were
marked "Confidential" not because Zonolite or Grace officials
pressured him to do so; it was simply the norm. State law required
him to inform only the company of his findings.

Wake's final correspondence with Grace is dated June 23, 1972,
in which he gave a brief nod of approval to the company's plans to
build a new mill at the mine, replacing the dry mill he'd been complaining about for the past sixteen years. After Wake's departure

and the construction of the new mill, the health department's communications with Grace took on a decidedly accommodating tone. In the state's first inspection of the new facilities in 1974, engineer Robert Hill found that one-third of the samples he took from the new mill and 11 percent of those from the new screening plant still exceeded existing limits for asbestos, and half of the rest broke new levels being proposed by the fledging federal EPA. Hill, nonetheless, was pleased with these results. Unlike Wake, he made no specific recommendations for bringing Grace into compliance, but left it up to the company's discretion: "In summary these samples indicate that the new process and equipment is achieving good control of airborne asbestos in most areas. They also point out several areas where improvements could be made and significant long-term benefits achieved. ...

"I sincerely appreciated the cooperation and assistance provided by you and your staff during this survey. While this survey was made at an inopportune time for you, we are now satisfied that the new process and plant has significantly improved working conditions. At some time in the future, after operation of the new plant has stabilized, I would like to collect a series of personal samples to verify that employee exposures to asbestos remain acceptable."

It is telling of Montana's attitude toward mining regulations that a state engineer found it "acceptable" for Grace to consistently overexpose its workers to asbestos. But at least in 1974 the state was making an effort to keep track of the doings up in Libby. After Hill's report, it would be seven years before another state inspector traveled to Libby. Pat Driscoll, a Montana Tech grad with a degree in environmental engineering, pulled the job of inspecting the mine from 1981 to 1987 for the Department of Health, and his authority was narrow. His job was to enforce the state's air quality standards, which meant the air the public was breathing. The miners' health was an occupational issue, and out of his reach. "I was well aware that that mine, in processing vermiculite, had a lot of tremolite asbestos associated with it, and that at least at that point in time there had been a significant occupational exposure to asbestos," he admits. "Neither our agency nor EPA, for that matter, has occupational regulatory authority. I don't say that as a cop-out or to lay the blame. That's just strictly our only authority: ambient air, that is, where the public has access. That's where the standards apply."

During Driscoll's tenure as inspector, the state continued its accommodating tone. On January 31, 1984, Department of Health supervisor Bob Raish wrote Earl Lovick a month ahead of the state's visit to let the company know when the state would be sending inspectors to collect samples of particulate matter in the air. Grace responded by sending its own samples to the agency before the state's inspectors could get there. Driscoll says he did inspect the mine later that year in June, but the subject of asbestos never came up. His 1985 and 1987 inspections were hampered by the fact that the mill was closed down on the days he was there to take samples. Driscoll says that in 1987 he asked the company to share their own data on asbestos emissions. The company's environmental specialist said he'd have to check with corporate headquarters before releasing that kind of information. It was never forthcoming. "My request for monitoring data during my site inspection on September 17, 1987 was specific to their in-plant asbestos testing for occupational exposure which did not fall within our regulatory purview," Driscoll wrote me to clarify the situation. "I do know that I never received any data from Mr. Jacobs but I do not recall if he ever got back to me specifically stating a corporate decision on providing the data. Later in 1987 or early 1988, my job duties were changed and inspection responsibilities at the site were assigned to another inspector. In reviewing the files, it does not appear that any occupational monitoring data was ever submitted by the company."

And finally the state had—and still has—no regulations specific to ambient asbestos in the air. "It's like saying people shouldn't drive fast, but never setting a speed limit. What does that really mean and how do you really regulate it?" Driscoll says, referring to Montana's brief flirtation with an undefined statewide "reasonable and prudent" speed limit. "That's where it's still at: there still is no ambient air quality standard for asbestos. So it would have been hard even if we had tried to pursue it as a public health issue then. It would have been difficult to say how much is too much."

Don Judge, former director of the state's AFL-CIO, says it's not clear that current state law would protect workers from another Libby. "There's clearly a problem when an agency finds a hazard in the workplace and its response is to inform management, not the workers," he says. "There is a right to know law in this state, but it applies to chemicals. I don't know if asbestos would fit the definition of a chemical.

"This sort of thing happens all over the world. It's more difficult in the U.S. now because the workforce is more sophisticated and communities are more involved in protecting themselves. Is it going to happen again in Libby, Montana? I doubt it. But clearly, if you wanted to pack up a Zonolite or asbestos operation and move it someplace like Venezuela or Argentina, it could happen easily."

Driscoll says he finds it curious that so many people now say they knew nothing about the asbestos problems in Libby. He recalls extensive discussions of the matter as part of his course work at Montana Tech. "There was lots of discussion about the asbestos issues in general, but specifically at that mine. That's one of the things that's always confused me a little about now—the perception that no one knew of this issue when it was certainly discussed at length."

Driscoll is partly right; people at all levels of government knew there was an asbestos problem in Libby. But only Grace saw the big picture. The situation was a little like a crooked game of cards: Grace had marked the deck and hidden a few aces under the table. Only those in management knew all the facts. Grace had the X rays, and company officials chronicled their deathwatch in a series of macabre internal memos, noting as each man's health declined on the grainy black-and-white film. Local doctors were at the company's beck and call, while outside health officials had to beg for scraps of data that were never forthcoming. Grace had read the 1977 hamster study and knew its results boded ill not just for the health of anyone who came in contact with their tremolite fiber, but also for the mine's financial future. By the time Driscoll made his first inspection, Grace had amassed a collection of death certificates and could call upon two decades' worth of detailed asbestos fiber counts. But they weren't sharing.

Adding to the confusion, each agency played by a different set of rules: Congress charged the Occupational Health and Safety Administration with setting asbestos standards, but enforcement was confined to the federal Bureau of Mines and its successors. The EPA and state could assert authority if there was a general health hazard, but couldn't set foot past that boundary. The resulting regulatory scheme was a disjointed mess.

THERE ARE THOSE WHO will argue that setting the U.S. Bureau of Mines to regulate the mining industry is akin to letting NASCAR drivers enforce the speed limit. The agency's original mandate was a lesson in conflicts of interest: the bureau was charged both with enforcing mining regulations and with "resource development," acting as a booster for the industry. While Congress attempted to fix the problem with the establishment of a separate enforcement branch of the bureau in 1973, the reputation stuck. But for all the criticism of the bureau—deserved or not—it was the only agency paying any attention to Grace's mine in Libby for most of the 1970s.

The bureau's initial inspection in 1971 gave the feds their first indication that there was an asbestos problem in Libby, Montana. The old dry mill was still operating, so the results of that inspection provided a set of benchmark readings that various agencies would use to guess at the nature of the exposure-disease relationship for the next three decades. The bureau's inspectors counted asbestos particles in the air ranging from 13 to 71 fibers/ml (by this time, scientists could count the exact asbestos bodies, a figure expressed in fibers per milliliter of sampled air). The industry had set informal limits on asbestos exposure for itself at 5 fibers/ml in 1967, based on recommendations by the American Conference of Governmental Hygienists. The government was considering codifying that standard in 1971 as the "threshold limit value," or TLV. Behind the statistics were the men the bureau's inspectors encountered:

On a time-weighted-average basis, the top-floor operator was exposed to seven times the proposed TLV. He was required to wear a respirator on all but the first floor of the mill, or practically all the shift. The bottom-floor operator was exposed to seven times the proposed TLV. He was required to wear a respirator on all but the first floor of the mill, and despite his title, this meant practically all shift. The first floor presumably was relatively dust-free, but observation and the single area sample and office and lunch-room samples indicated that the first floor was dusty.

Two sweepers were sampled; both were exposed to seven times the proposed TLV. They were required to wear respirators in the dry mill in all but the first floor. During the sweeping and cleanup process, the settled dust, while being swept, fell through cracks in the floor and added to the ambient dust load in the air.

The tails-belt operator spent his time on the first floor where no respirator was required. Much of his duties involved working with wet muck in a wet area. Nevertheless his time-weighted average exposure was more than double the proposed TLV.

It goes on. The electrician received a dose of asbestos fiber of six times the allowable amount; the loading dock foreman's exposure was so high that it couldn't be quantified. The agency even sampled the bus that ferried the men back to town after their shift, and counted 1.7 fibers/ml.

In 1978, a new arm of the bureau, the Mine Safety and Health Administration (MSHA), took over inspection responsibilities. This agency did its job regularly and fulfilled each of its statutory responsibilities faithfully, according to an investigation by the Office of Inspector General in 2001. Yet the death toll mounted. "We do not believe that more inspections or sampling would have prevented the current situation in Libby," the Inspector General concluded. The system itself was broken.

First, former Grace employees told the Inspector General that the company often had advance notice of inspections. "Several interviewees stated that there were several 'signs' of an imminent inspection: the water truck would appear and begin watering down the dust; work assignments would be altered to allow for clean up, particularly with regard to potential safety violations; and MSHA

Inspectors normally checked into one of the three local motels in Libby the night prior to the inspection, allowing for the information to be spread by the townspeople."

Second, the Inspector General concluded that the legal limits for asbestos exposure weren't strict enough. "With few exceptions, laboratory analysis of the asbestos samples taken by MSHA Inspectors from 1978 through 1990 showed the samples to be under MSHA's regulated Permissible Exposure Limits (PEL). Yet a large number of former Grace employees and family members in Libby have contracted asbestos-related illness."

Third, the agency had no authority to address the issue of take-home contamination. And finally, the report concluded, the method of analysis used by almost everyone—looking for fibers with phase contrast microscopy—was woefully inadequate. In other words, MSHA enforced the letter of the law in Libby, but left its spirit to languish.

MEANWHILE, 2,000 miles to the east, a health crisis erupted at a Marysville, Ohio, company when four of its employees were diagnosed with bloody pleural effusions. O.M. Scott and Sons—now called the Scotts Company—makes some of the nation's most popular lawn and garden chemicals: Turf Builder, Miracle Gro, Roundup. In 1978 the four men, workers at Scott, had somehow developed holes in the delicate membranes around their lungs, and Scott officials were rightfully concerned. There in Marysville, Libby's EPA team leader Paul Peronard tells me, the federal regulatory system worked. Had the Grace corporation not stalled, the system might have worked in Libby, too.

The way U.S. law is set up, federal agencies rely on the candor of the industries they regulate both for setting health standards and for ferreting out problems. When the Scotts Company came up with four sick workers, its officials contacted the feds immediately. "Some information relating to one of our chemical fertilizer Plants has come to the attention of Scott which may or may not be reportable under the various statutes administered by your respective agencies," the Scotts attorney wrote to the EPA and federal

Occupational Safety and Health Administration. "We have resolved any doubt on this question by this letter in an effort to fully
advise you and seek your cooperation in dealing with the matter."
   The attorney went on to report that Scotts could not find any
material linking bloody pleural effusions to asbestos exposure, and
added that the people in its employ were exposed to levels of asbestos allowable within the law.

> We have no reason to believe our current Plant situation presents
> any risk of asbestos-related problems since it is in compliance with
> OSHA asbestos standards. Based on the low levels of fibers
> reported in our Plant at this time, the physicians involved have
> advised us that these findings do not indicate a current asbestos
> hazard to our workers, if in fact the effusions are related to the
> occupational exposures at Scott at all.
>   In summary, the situation present is a perplexing problem.
> There is no medical evidence or literature indicating these four
> cases are due to occupational exposures in the Scott Plant. Yet, the
> fact remains a cluster of four cases of this type would not be
> expected to be found in a much larger population than Scott's
> 500–600 workforce. Adding to this uncertainty is the fact that this
> condition has apparently arisen several years after plant exposure,
> but not within the expected timing of asbestos-like problems.

It has become a familiar chorus over the last several years: the
idea that because a company's asbestos levels are within the limits
set by the federal government, there shouldn't be any sick workers. And yet here they are: the irrefutable proof of gravestones and
oxygen tanks. The limits were wrong.
   At Scotts, officials from OSHA came in and did some testing,
and found that the company's health problems were much more
extensive than Scotts had realized. There were in fact nearly three
dozen workers with some kind of pleural disease, out of 125 tested.
But as to the cause, OSHA shrugged its shoulders. So Scotts
officials hired scientists from the University of Cincinnati to look
at the problem. Jim Lockey was just a grad student in those days,
looking for a thesis topic. He signed on to the project with his
professor, Dr. Stuart Brooks, and their research eventually linked

the illnesses to asbestos in the vermiculite Scotts used as an inert carrier for its chemicals.

The connection was not immediately obvious, Lockey says, because all kinds of things cause bloody pleural effusions. "There could have been an infectious cause, there could have been a viral cause, something like that. Chest trauma—you fracture a rib, you bleed into your chest. Certain types of pneumonia, cancer, can cause bloody pleural effusions." Once these were ruled out, the doctors took a look at the plant's industrial hygiene data, which included the information that the sacks of vermiculite from Libby were contaminated with asbestos. "That's not something that we see a lot of with asbestos exposure—it's an uncommon manifestation of asbestosis," he says. "If you have somebody who's had an occupational exposure to asbestos and they have a bloody pleural effusion, and you've ruled out all those other things I've just talked about, then you [are] into the category where it's most likely caused by asbestos exposure.

"And then we said we think this is probably related to asbestos. I think that's when the bells went off that there is something going on here," Lockey says. The Cincinnati scientists recommended that Scotts switch ore sources, and the company did so in 1980. The company had been getting half of its vermiculite from Libby and half from a mine in South Africa. After Lockey's study, the company began using ore from Grace's other vermiculite mine in South Carolina. Later, Lockey compared the asbestiforms from all three mines, as well as from one in Virginia, which together comprised 90 percent of the world's vermiculite source. Libby's ore, the scientists concluded, appeared to be the most dangerous, and the single difference was the "aspect ratio" of each fiber's length and width. In other words, Libby's fibers are long and narrow, spears that dig into lung tissue, while asbestos from the other mines tended toward the geometric equivalent of obesity.

As the revelations from the Scotts Company made the rounds in federal circles, suddenly everyone was interested in Libby. The National Institute of Occupational Safety and Health was the first agency to approach Grace after the news broke, and expressed interest in doing a study of Libby workers. Company officials met twice with NIOSH representatives in November 1980. At the first meeting, Grace officials gave NIOSH agents only the most vague data about their operations. Undeterred, the NIOSH people sat down with Grace officials a few weeks later and pushed their position more forcefully, informing the company that they would do a comprehensive epidemiological study of Libby's miners in 1981.

First, Grace officials tried to diffuse the situation by clouding the issue of the company's culpability for the Scott situation. According to a corporate memo summarizing the talk, they told the NIOSH representatives, "this study could create a lot of loose talk with serious implications and have a deleterious, unjustified and pointless impact on Grace's vermiculite business. [Harry] Borgstedt stated a viral infection was a more likely Scott explanation than vermiculite. [Safety Director Harry] Eschenbach stated that chemicals handled and applied at Scott were further suspects."

The NIOSH people, however, were well prepared to be stalled. When the agency's epidemiologist asked Grace for the company's data on each employee's exposure history, Grace officials equivocated: "When we indicated this would be difficult and subjective, she [the epidemiologist] produced a 1968/69 Earl Lovick summary which did this." The meeting was a stalemate and ended rather abruptly.

Dr. John Dement, NIOSH team leader on the project, recalls that Grace had no interest in cooperating. "They were dragging their feet," he says. "They had a strategy that they had pretty well thought through. They were resistant to the study, and that's pretty well summed up in the memos, which I saw many years later."

The memos Dement refers to are straightforward in their intent. In one, a Grace official wrote in the margins that Dement "was a real problem: wise, somewhat nasty ..." Another memo, penned by Grace executive Robert Locke, outlines the company's strategy. He listed their options as:

> a) Obstruct and block, possibly even contesting in the courts. As I understand it, we'd lose and this is not exactly the image we try to project.

b) Be slow, review things extensively and contribute to delay. This might not be bad policy generally and it is possible that the new Administration's policies will make NIOSH more selective in how scarce staff resources are allocated after January 20, 1981.

c) Publish a "pre-emptive epidemiological study." This could attenuate the resume-enhancing potential for NIOSH study personnel. This could also be a checkpoint for a subsequent NIOSH study when it is released.

d) Cooperate fully. This agency and its personnel have not always acted with high levels of professionalism on past studies. This option would save NIOSH time and effort, make their study more comprehensive and possibly rule out some inaccuracies. It would not necessarily make NIOSH's conclusions any more responsible.

e) Actively go upstream in NIOSH to personally repeat the same arguments, the first time immediately after receipt of the protocol.

f) Actively seek to turn off the sources of the pressure for the study by personally repeating the same arguments. However, the sources may have supplementary reasons not fully shared by NIOSH.

g) Attempt to apply influence via congressmen, senators, lobbyists or others to get it turned off. This might result in delay without turning it off. However, it is not necessarily successful, can backfire and to be effective must be developed over long periods of time due to the trust required.

In the end, Grace appears to have attacked the NIOSH problem on several fronts. In one letter, NIOSH reports that Grace attorney Mario Favorito threatened to "present its position on this study to 'higher government authority,'" namely the secretary of the Department of Labor. Grace also seems to have gone for option c: the company commissioned its own study in the form of hiring researchers from McGill University in Montreal. (These researchers, who published their findings in the 1985 *British Journal of Industrial Medicine*, found not only that Libby's miners had an excessively high mortality rate from respiratory disease, they also pronounced the lung cancer rate to be higher than that found in commercial chrysotile asbestos miners.)

When Locke referred to the likelihood that scarce NIOSH staff resources would be reallocated after January 21, 1981, more than idle speculation was involved. Ronald Reagan was sworn into office that day after winning the presidency on a platform of shrinking the size of the federal government. To work toward that end, he appointed his friend J. Peter Grace, CEO of the Grace corporation, to head up a committee that would search out waste in government and cut bureaucracy down to size. No evidence has come to light that the Grace Commission interfered with the NIOSH study, though the implication of the Grace corporation's influence must have been clear to everyone involved.

Former union president Bob Wilkins says he remembers the situation well. "First off I got a call from a Dr. Banks, and he was with NIOSH, so he wanted to know if my employees, the union members, would work with them in an inspection of the work site. And I assured him that we would, because we wanted to have a clean and safe environment to work in. So he said, all right. His intentions were that he would bring in like a trailer with a lab on it, and he would have five technicians, and they would set up on campsite, and work the area that our people was working in. And I said sure, we'll cooperate with you one hundred percent on that. Well, he was setting up everything to come in here. Well, as soon as he notified W.R. Grace, the shit hit the fan then."

NIOSH sent Wilkins copies of all the correspondence between Grace and the agency so the union would know what was going on. He was cynically amused by the whole thing, but expected the government would get its way. Then the bottom dropped out.

"There was one paragraph in the letter that really caught my attention, and that was something to the effect that, if you didn't call this study off, they would use their influence in Washington, D.C. Now when that came out, that really got me because Peter Grace had just been appointed by President Reagan to head up the Grace Commission, and it consisted of about twenty-five to thirty high top officials throughout the United States on ways of downsizing the government. So here we got Peter Grace sitting on the right hand of Reagan. ...

"Shortly after that, Banks called me and told me, we won't be coming to Libby. The project's been called off. I'm being transferred to another department. I said well, I'm sorry to hear that. Well, that was the end of Dr. Banks. Never heard anything more about him."

In fact the study was completed, though it was later than the agency had planned. And the results—published in 1987—were handicapped by the fact that Grace did not share its X rays with the government, nor did they reveal that a hamster study of Libby's tremolite fiber had been conducted in 1977 and had revealed Libby's specific asbestos fiber to be a particularly virulent cause of cancer and respiratory disease.

At about the same time NIOSH was haggling over its intentions to do an epidemiological study, the EPA announced its intention to complete a sweeping survey of the vermiculite industry, focusing on rumors of a connection to asbestos-related diseases. Prodded by reports of illness at the Scott plant in Ohio and bolstered with the Bureau of Mines' 1971 report on the existence of asbestos in the Libby ore, the EPA wrote in a June 1980 assessment, "the extent of exposure from vermiculite derived from the Libby mine is likely to be large, considering that this source accounts for approximately 80% of the vermiculite used in the U.S." The agency declared its intention to study the industry of vermiculite mining and processing, starting with W.R. Grace's Libby operations, and to investigate the possibility of consumer exposure to asbestos from vermiculite products like insulation and lawn care materials.

The EPA had even sent a team to Libby to take samples at the end of October 1980, and to Grace's other vermiculite mine in South Carolina a week later, when the plug was pulled abruptly on that study as well. The agency released a report in 1982 explaining the aborted effort: "The original scope of the study included two phases. The first phase was the collection and analysis of air and bulk samples associated with vermiculite ore and beneficiated vermiculite from the four major U.S. mines and ports of entry. The second phase was for a similar effort for a representative number of exfoliation plants.

"Because of priority shifts within EPA, the second phase was not undertaken and the scope of the first phase was reduced," the report's author explained dryly.

Twenty years later, the EPA's Paul Peronard notes the irony. "That was probably the euphemism of the day. They did a fraction of the work that they had planned to do," he says. "What's amazing to me is if you look at the tenor of the reports—like if you start with the investigation they were doing at the O.M. Scott plant in Marysville, Ohio. There was a ... notification that O.M. Scott made to the EPA under the TSCA law—and basically TSCA's the Toxic Substances Control Act. And it says, 'Hey look, if a company encounters a substance that they know is causing health problems, they gotta notify the EPA.' It's fairly straightforward. So O.M. Scott does this in 1978 and there's actually a whole series of reports about Marysville, Ohio, where they figure out that the problem is the asbestos in the Libby ore. That's what prompted the investigations in 1980. If you look at some of the background documents, people were treating it as an awful big deal. And then it just stops. There was no grand explanation as to why that should be the case."

Except, he agrees, for the concurrence of Ronald Reagan's election and J. Peter Grace's new position of authority in the Reagan administration. "Do I have any proof or evidence of that? No, not really," he admits. "They were clever enough not to write anything down, I guess. But you know the timing surely is a grand coincidence if that's the case."

In any case, EPA investigators made no more visits to Libby after the November election. Air samples taken during those single trips to Libby and Enoree, South Carolina (both during rainy weeks when the dust conditions were at their lowest), originally were to be analyzed by the more accurate—and expensive—electron microscope. Instead the agency relied on the old phase contrast microscope, missing the bulk of asbestos fibers in the air.

In the wake of the scandal in 1999, the Office of Inspector General would investigate the EPA's actions during the early 1980s. In that report the OIG concluded that a pitiful lack of communication was at fault for the agency's failure to follow through on the clear threat to people's health. Whether Reagan's Grace Commission had a hand in the situation or not, Peronard says that he blames his agency. And that knowledge has left him fighting cynicism.

"I think less of my agency, I guess, than when I started. Even the progress we made in Libby since we started in '99, you know— we've made it very hard to get things done up there. People seem more concerned about the politics and the precedents: the decision, for example, on the insulation removal. People are more concerned with—well, we might have to do something across the country with other insulation in other places—than they are about the fact that this stuff's not safe. I guess the only thing I always keep in my mind is that if you don't keep plugging at it, then it just simply won't get done. I mean, we have made a whole bunch of progress in Libby. If I allowed myself just to get in a bitch-and-moan operation, we wouldn't get stuff done."

In fact, anyone in a position of authority at the EPA could have taken on the mantle Peronard assumed when his bosses sent him to Libby just before Christmas in 1999, and they didn't. I ask him why, and he gives a typical Peronardian answer, the sort that makes the press swoon for him. "Um, because we're a bunch of chicken-shits? You know, it's not that dorky of a question. It's actually one I really hoped the IG investigation would have looked at a little harder. There's no real good reason for why we didn't do more.

"If you look at the timing, the agency had started sort of divesting itself of asbestos programs and regulations starting in the early to mid-'80s. This is something that was much more complicated. Almost all asbestos regulation was set on products that were specifically made with an asbestos content, chrysotile asbestos. It's what all the microscope, analytical techniques were geared toward, and this was sort of an oddball. It was a tramp contaminant that nobody really thought was making it into the final consumer products. So I guess from the EPA, everybody was just saying, 'It's a mine worker problem, it's not our business, and we don't think it's causing much of a problem elsewhere.' We were fairly content to accept that answer."

IN CONTRAST TO PERONARD, state EPA chief John Wardell is
a fairly typical bureaucrat. He has answers to only the most innocuous questions, and really thinks my time would be better
spent investigating other agencies, like the Bureau of Mines or the
federal Occupational Safety and Health Administration. But in
fact, his Helena office was tipped off once in 1984 and twice in the
mid-1990s to the likelihood of an asbestos problem at the old
Grace mine. In 1994, Wardell's boss, EPA regional director Bill
Yellowtail, won one of the largest asbestos-related settlements in
the country—$510,000—when Grace spent a year and a half de-
molishing five asbestos-contaminated buildings at the old mine
taking practically none of the precautions required by law. The
agency wouldn't have even known about the demolition if a Libby
resident hadn't tipped them off.

No matter how I press, Wardell can't remember any details of
his dealings with Grace, though he has worked in this office since
1983. He passes me off to Betsy Wahl, one of his employees, who
is charged with managing the air compliance program. Wahl has
only been working at the state EPA since 1997, and while she has
all of her predecessors' records at her disposal, she says that for
Libby this amounts to one thin file. "It's kind of a puzzle—different agencies deal with different aspects," she says. "We dealt with
the structures, and if it had been an asbestos mine, we would have
regulated it. But since it was a vermiculite mine contaminated
with asbestos, it's just an odd deal. A very unfortunate odd deal."
Unlike Wardell, Wahl really wants to help me, giving me a name
and toll-free number for someone in the Denver office who might
shed some light on the matter. She promises to look back over the
file again, a task performed exhaustively a year ago when the federal Inspector General's office sent investigators to Montana to
find out why the EPA never did anything about the asbestos problem in Libby. But she tells me not to hope for too much. As the
only EPA employee in the state working on air quality, she says she
spends her time trying to cover mines that are still in operation.
She suspects the same was true of her predecessors. Too few resources spread too thin to do the job thoroughly.

WHEN GOVERNOR MARC RACICOT stepped to the podium that damp December night in 1999, he represented to Libby all the bureaucrats who had ignored them. He inherited the legacy of mistakes dating back to before he was even born. And more hung on Racicot's presentation at the meeting that night than his public image in Montana. A presidential election was on, and Racicot was rumored to be in line for a cabinet seat, most likely as attorney general or heading up the Interior Department for George W. Bush (a post for which he later took himself out of the running). In fact, the Montana governor skipped a similar meeting in Libby just after the story broke, opting instead to help his Texan counterpart prepare for a debate in New Hampshire. Scrutinized by Bush's people on one side and Montanans on the other, Racicot would have to muster all his political skills for the evening's performance.

By all accounts, Marc Racicot has considerable skills to draw upon. "Racicot has proven to be one of the most popular governors in the history of the state," gushed historian Michael Malone in his 1996 book, *Montana: A Contemporary Profile.* "Clean cut and handsome, articulate, engaging and radiating sincerity and integrity—in fact, his poll popularity ratings routinely surpass 70 percent." The governor won reelection handily in 1996, arguably because his opponent, Chuck Blaylock, died a few weeks before the vote. Yet there is no indication that Blaylock, a loyal Democrat who ran mainly out of a sense of duty when his own party failed to mount a serious challenge to Racicot, would have done any better had he lived. When Blaylock stepped to the plate as a matter of principle, Racicot's Republicans held a strong majority in the legislature, and Democrats were losing ground in their traditional power bases of Missoula, Butte, and along the Hi-Line farming communities. The governor barely needed to campaign.

The only crack in Racicot's facade appeared over time, like concrete frozen and thawed repeatedly over too many years exposed to the elements. Racicot inherited a policy of killing wild bison who wandered beyond the boundaries of Yellowstone National Park. Each winter the governor continued, defended, and at times escalated the slaughter, insisting the policy was a matter of concern about disease and cattle. In fact, Montana was fighting a range war, the old battle for control over the state's vast public lands. But the nuances of western environmental policies were lost on the national audience that tuned in to the killing fields, and when nearly 1,200 buffalo were gunned down by state agents in the winter of 1996–97, Racicot's Reaganesque image suffered repeated blows.

Now adding pressure to these cracks was a plague in his native Libby. Pundits liked to compare Racicot's charisma to former president Ronald Reagan's Teflon, but the people in this relatively conservative community were beginning to see things differently. "Better hold on to your seat or he'll blow sunshine up your you-know-what," Les Skramstad jokes as we file in for the town meeting.

Regardless of Racicot's shortcomings, it is still a hometown crowd that has gathered to grill the governor, and just a week before Christmas, they are inclined to be generous. Racicot has little difficulty warming up the room, drawing on memories common to many of those in attendance. He begins by talking of his childhood in Libby. "I remember moving what appeared to be giant bags of Zonolite into our house; they were very light so that a small person such as myself could move them. I remember putting them into the attic and walls of our home, and emptying them into the garden." Racicot recalls playing at the baseball field near Zonolite's expansion plant and swinging on a rope and dropping into the piles of vermiculite, just as all the other kids did.

The reporters in attendance (including a woman from Anaconda's old newspaper chain, still a virtual monopoly owned by the Iowa-based Lee Enterprises) want to know who is responsible—the old "who knew what, when?" But to Libby residents, this meeting isn't about telling a compelling story; it's a matter of life and death, and their questions reflect the difference.

A burly, flannel-shirted man stands in the bleachers and asks, "How much of it do you have to breathe for it to kill you?"

That's one for the state's medical officer, Dr. Michael Spence. "I don't know. I don't think anybody knows," he says. "Two individuals exposed to the same level of fibers will react differently."

There's a long pause. This is not the answer anyone expected. The local county sanitarian has been quoted of late saying that there is less than 1 percent asbestos content in the town's air, and that level is perfectly safe. No one is sure where he came up with this idea, but the business community latched on to it. This statement is repeated in the cafes and bars as gospel. Dr. Spence is now blaspheming the Chamber of Commerce line.

The heavyset man works to get his mind around the next question: "Then how do we know what percentage is safe?"

The answer, Spence admits, is that you don't. "That 1 percent figure does not address the issue of what you breathe into your lungs. With inhalation, you get sick two ways, there are two possible outcomes. Asbestosis—typically it takes longer doses over time, it wears out your lungs over time. With mesothelioma, it takes lower doses; we don't see that happen as often.

"There's a long latency period for both. Usually we see asbestosis in miners, but apparently we're seeing asbestosis in nonminers too."

That is the crux of the matter. As the agency's toxicologist, Chris Weis, told me earlier in the day, unless there is some threat to the health of the public at large, the EPA has no authority. When only miners were getting sick, it was none of their concern: "The EPA doesn't have the authority or responsibility for occupational safety," he said. "That's NIOSH or OSHA."

By early 2000, Peronard would report that his agency had counted forty cases of nonoccupational asbestos-related illness attributable to the mine at Libby, a distinction that became meaningless as the feds eventually identified eighteen pathways of exposure in the community. But as of Christmas 1999, asbestosis is still a miners' disease to this crowd. People are worried about the economic fallout, and in response the EPA has set up an extensive air and soil testing plan.

"We're doing only surface samples on driveways and yards to see what gets kicked up into the air from normal activity," Peronard says. "We're doing 2-foot core samples in gardens, the ball fields, places where there historically were piles of it."

Which begs the question: "What will happen if you find it deep in there?" Libby is already reeling from declines in the logging industry and has been trying to rebuild itself as a tourist community, drawing travelers from nearby Glacier National Park to what's left of the national forests and admittedly picturesque but dammed-up rivers in the surrounding countryside. The state AFL-CIO director, Don Judge, has taken to calling Libby "America's Chernobyl," a tourism buzz-kill if ever there was one.

Unlike the radioactive legacy at the infamous nuke plant, asbestos is relatively easy to deal with. "We'll either bury it here or haul it somewhere else and bury it," Peronard says. "Let's do a for-instance. If we found it in the ball field, typically what we'd do is restrict further development. You couldn't put a basement in there, or you could if it were completely enclosed."

As the evening wears on, the crowd tires. The annual bout of flu has turned up early this year, and I can only imagine how it is for those in the audience trailing oxygen tanks, for whom even minor pulmonary infections can mean dire consequences. Even those with mild asbestosis could be one cold away from needing oxygen themselves. It's time to wrap things up, and Peronard obliges.

He tells the crowd that his agency will try to set up programs and protocols that will continue long after the EPA crowd goes back to Denver. "There are medical questions as well as where the stuff is. With building codes, we can set it up so asbestos inspections are mandatory when you're remodeling. Same with local doctors—we want them to be able to do X-ray and pulmonary exams. That way, when the federal government goes home, we leave behind someone to keep up with that."

A final question remains, and a man on the far side of the gym stands to ask it. "How can we trust you?"

It's Peronard's turn to pause. "You mean, in the past you've been assured that things were safe, and given the latency of the disease, how do you know twenty years from now we haven't sold you a bill of goods?"

There is an interested silence as Peronard, head down, considers his answer. Looking up again, he addresses the audience with conviction.

"I promise you we probably won't find all of it. We will find the vast majority and, depending on what's called for, clean it up or not. But it will be on file for you in the future. To the broader question of how can you trust us, in the past you've dealt with government as a broad, faceless bureaucracy. Your satisfaction or not is my responsibility. I'm accountable for how this information is tracked." During the past three decades, no one in government who knew about the asbestos problem had stepped in and made it their personal responsibility to protect Libby's workers. During the past few weeks, after the story broke in a Seattle newspaper, most of the state's politicians and bureaucrats alike fled from the scandal, while a few others stood on the sidelines saying, "I told you so."

Governor Racicot refuses to assign culpability to anyone, and rebuffs those looking for a place to lay blame, in particular exonerating the state for its tragic inattention to Libby. "There is some surprise associated with what we're talking about this evening," he tells the crowd. "Quite frankly, over all these years, I've never had a single conversation about an existing public health problem, or the possibility of a threat to the health of people in Libby. There's been some concern about reports that were kept confidential. As all of us know, the facts and circumstances have changed over the last several decades. Many things occurred in the 1950s and '60s, even in the '70s, that would not occur in this day and age." Given one last chance to lead his people, to face the wrongs of the last century and help right them, Governor Racicot instead has chosen a political route.

He is not alone. In the past few weeks since the story broke, no one in a position of power in Montana has accepted blame for anything.

Only Peronard has faced it and spoken the whole truth, and with that simple act, he has begun to win Libby's trust.

AS THE TOWN GRUDGINGLY ACCEPTED the EPA's help—largely on the promise of a young man who showed the potential of great character—Libby made a turn onto a path away from all the darkness in its past, knowing only that there would be more pain and death in the future, but hoping for something better. But as Libby's long nightmare began to fade, Grace's legacy refused to quit the world. Among the nation's estimated 12 to 35 million buildings with Libby's insulation were two towers once prominent in the New York skyline. When the World Trade Center was being constructed, Grace sold its contractors thousands of tons of ore to fireproof the outside columns of the giant buildings. On September 11, 2001, the jet-fueled attacks of terrorists unleashed a time bomb of unthinkable proportions.

A Miner's Wife

Ryan Bundrock seems to believe he is immortal. He clings to this belief, say his family and acquaintances, despite strong evidence to the contrary: he has been diagnosed with asbestosis. But only rock stars burn out so fast and die so young. At twenty-one, he can't admit to his disease, and won't talk about it with outsiders. So his grandmother talks for him.

Sorrow is the bottomless well at the center of Helen Bundrock's life, and her tears flow from it freely and often. It is as if she were given a choice between anger and grief, and chose the latter. "Anger will kill you. It will eat you up faster than anything," she says. Helen has reason for both: the seventy-year-old, born in South Dakota and raised in Kalispell, will likely lose most of her family to Grace's asbestosis. She is sick with it and is on oxygen. She buried her husband, Art, who died of heart failure brought on by the strain of breathing through asbestos-damaged lungs in 1998, after nineteen years on the job for W.R. Grace. In addition to her grandson Ryan, four of her five children have been diagnosed with the disease.

The tears come as she flips through a family photo album. There's her handsome son Bill, a strong face, mustache, and brown eyes. "Our family's doctor's wife called. She said, 'He's the most handsome man I've ever seen,'" she says. And Art, in this picture a slight man with a gray complexion, his eyes tight with pain, is wearing a brace. She starts to explain, through sobs that leave as fast as they come, that he broke his neck one day, having fallen down because he wasn't carrying his oxygen tank. "He hated that oxygen tank, really hated it. Because, you know, we would go back and forth to Arizona and it got to where he couldn't lift it," she says. "I could, yeah. But he hated to see me have to do that." Adding insult to injury, she says, Grace denied Art's pension one year after he died, after it was too late for her to do anything about it.

Helen has a large grandmother's laugh, a soft body made for comforting children, and a musical voice that bears surprisingly little animosity toward the Grace company and its people. She recalls a kindness Earl Lovick's wife, Bonnie, once committed: "I was a checker at a grocery store. She said, 'Helen, you look so sad.' I said, 'You know I am. I turned fifty today and nobody remembered.' And she went out and bought me some flowers." Her tears come again. "So there was good in both of them. I just feel bad, the whole thing that happened. You know and through it all, you know, like Earl and Paul Norris the CEO and all of them, I feel as sorry for them as I do for us, because we are not the final judge. They'll be judged for their actions and it won't be a nice sight."

Ryan stays with his grandmother off and on. He has worked as a miner and a forest firefighter, but started school at the University of Montana in the fall of 2001. Helen worries about him, but knows she can only do so much. "He did say last night, he said, 'You think I should go for the testing?' I said, 'Well, it's up to you. But I would if I were you. And get a baseline anyway so you know where it's going from there.'"

She sighs, and we sit in the silence of her living room, sealed against the summer heat by the air conditioner. "To me it's not going to be a bad thing to die," she says. "I don't know why I had to live all these years after Art died."

SEVEN

Wages of Greed

SEPTEMBER 26, 2001, is a strikingly pretty day in northwestern Montana, and for the first time in weeks it seems fitting to celebrate. The rich, deep hues provoked by autumn's diffuse sunlight exorcise the pall cast by the month's events in New York City, at least in this corner of the world. It's Gayla Benefield's birthday next week, so her kids are throwing a surprise party just outside of town at the steakhouse where her daughter Julie works. She had been on her way to an economic development meeting that night, but the ruse—that Julie had a migraine and wanted her mother— worked. Everyone shouts at the appropriate moment, and if Gayla isn't surprised, she's gracious enough not to show it.

The crowd is a mix of family, friends, and asbestos campaigners: Les and Norita Skramstad, of course; Jenan Swenson's former in-laws, Carrie and Robert Dedrick; Gayla's sister Eva, her accountant, her lawyer. The EPA guys were supposed to show up too, but were distracted by a tire fire south of Polson on their way to the party. Attorney Roger Sullivan, ever neurotic, asks if the festivities are going to be on the record. We haggle a bit and I offer to use discretion. It really isn't needed—the toasts and roasts are all good-natured. Norita passes on the microphone, so Les gets up first to tell about the time he and Gayla traveled to Washington, D.C., to testify against a bill that would have effectively cancelled most Libby claimants' rights to go to court. Wanting a beer one night, they walked endlessly looking for a bar; the one they found had never heard of go-cups (a Montana standard, for those who literally want "one for the road").

When Roger's turn comes, he talks of the difficulty of working for a woman who knows her mind and speaks it freely. A few weeks back, for instance, he picked up the alternative weekly newspaper from Missoula and read the first sentence of the cover story: "When it comes to her feelings about Governor Judy Martz, 62-year-old grandmother Gayla Benefield doesn't mince words. 'She's about ready to get a letter from me saying, 'Fuck you.'"

"I didn't say that," Gayla deadpans. And she's fifty-eight, thank you very much. Roger gets his next, as she makes fun of the way his "lawyer's butt" looks in a pair of jeans. The testimonials go on; Jenan (who had to cut back her cigarette ration to pay for her share of the party) forces a video camera in my hands when the adult kids stand up to eulogize the parent whose favorite saying seems to be "I brought you into this world, I can take you out of it." When Gayla's husband, David, takes the microphone, the jovial mood takes an earnest turn. He was asked recently, he says, if he had ever objected to Gayla's campaign against Grace, a hobby that turned their private lives public and their quiet community upside down. "She had that look in her eye," David says with a good-natured grin. "I knew better than to stand in her way." Then an older woman stands to make a toast: "If it weren't for Gayla, nobody would care about those poor people breathing asbestos back in New York."

It's been only a few weeks since the World Trade Center's collapse, and we're just now starting to hear rumors of high asbestos readings in the massive dust cloud that blanketed Lower Manhattan. EPA director Christine Todd Whitman has declared the area safe, but in fact both her agency and independent monitors have found the deadly fibers in the air, in the dust, in people's homes, and in their offices. According to the *New York Times*, approximately 20,000 people live within a half mile of the former World Trade Center. There is potentially a great tragedy in the making, the full scale of which perhaps can be understood only by the people gathered here tonight. There is silence, a collective shudder, at the thought of it.

Maybe, maybe. There are a lot of unanswered questions. But New York's EPA officials could have had a running start on the situation had they listened to their counterparts from Denver, much wiser after two years of dealing with the Libby mess. If the New York EPA had paid attention, they would have known that the old method of counting fibers is dreadfully inadequate, that people can get sick forty years after smaller, briefer exposures than were commonly accepted as safe, and that honesty and candor are the only way to earn the respect and cooperation of those you are trying to help.

Though none of us know it yet, the link from Libby to New York is closer than the commonality of death. According to the man who engineered the towers, W.R. Grace supplied the fireproofing that enveloped the steel beams holding the buildings up. And all the vermiculite in that material—thousands of tons' worth—came from the mine on Vermiculite Mountain.

But in the days and weeks after the terrorist attacks, the East Coast feds were more concerned with the panic that more bad news might bring, so even as Gayla was blowing out the candles on her cake, rescue crews were working around the clock in the dust without proper respirators. Within a few weeks, people would move back into their homes. Those with the foresight and money could have their apartments tested and cleaned. As for everyone else, they might as well be living in one of Libby's old houses, their apartments potentially just as full of invisible death as those Montana homes sifting Zonolite dust from the attic that only the fanciest wet HEPA vacuum can clean up.

Someone should have known better. Libby's EPA guys offered their expertise, their microscopes, the benefit of their experience, and were rebuffed. "We were not asked to participate in the response to the WTC disaster and we feel it would be inappropriate for us to second guess actions taken there since we are not apprised of all the variables," toxicologist Chris Weis e-mailed me. "Our responsibility and focus here in Denver is to assure that the people of Libby receive the best analysis, and public health response that we can provide."

One New Yorker, a woman named Elizabeth Berger, testified before a Senate subcommittee five months later on the difficulties and uncertainties facing the World Trade Center's former neighbors:

It took eight guys in white suits and respirators five days to clean my apartment. But is it clean? No one tells you what to keep and what to toss. ... What's in the stuff? Every day the air smelled different and the winds blew a different course.

We reluctantly made our own rules, divined from press reports, high school science as we remembered it and the advice of friends and neighbors. But even that was mixed. One scientist friend had his apartment tested and declared it safe for his family; the managing agent of his building, however, reported high levels of asbestos and lead. In the end, 248 stuffed animals, eight handmade baby quilts, five mattresses, a trousseau's worth of sheets and towels, a kitchen full of food and 13 leaf and lawn bags of toys went into our trash, but not our books, draperies and upholstered furniture or our clothes, though the bill to dry clean them industrially was $16,500. ... Some people we know repainted but kept their mattresses. Some people kept their stuffed animals but threw away their furniture. Some people kept what they couldn't bear to lose and got rid of the rest. We have still not decided what to do about our floors: Will stripping, sanding and resealing them contain the toxic mix of asbestos, fiberglass, concrete, human remains, heavy metals and the vague "particulates," or just release more of it into our indoor air?

Indoor air quality is a touchy issue in our building. Converted in the late 1970s, we have a primitive air system that circulates air from apartment to apartment. Some people in our building hired professional cleaners. Others did it themselves, and a few locked the door and didn't come back for a while. After the guys in the suits left, we sealed our windows, filtered our vents and bought six triple-HEPA-filtered air purifiers, which we run 24 hours a day. My clean air is making its way through the building, as is that of my less fastidious neighbors.

Berger's current troubles are rooted in events that took place more than twenty years before Osama bin Laden was born. The leaders of America's asbestos industry knew they were in trouble by the early 1930s, but through a convoluted web of secret research and linguistic and legal maneuvers, managed to stay solvent for another fifty years to keep their dirty secret quiet long enough to build the world's greatest skyscrapers, including the Twin Towers of New York.

Members of the asbestos industry collectively defined their difficulties in 1936, when approximately 250 people from fifty companies gathered at a conference sponsored by the Mellon Institute
of Industrial Research, based at the University of Pittsburgh, to
talk about dust problems. A representative from Johns-Manville
reported back on the proceedings.

> It appeared that among the problems common to all industries
> were the following:
>   (1) The menace of ambulance chasing lawyers in combination
> with unscrupulous doctors. The uncertainties surrounding the
> diagnosis of any of the various forms of pneumoconiosis are so
> many that a question of fact is presented in every case. Expert
> testimony can be produced by both plaintiff and defendant and it
> is for the jury to decide whose experts are correct in their inter-
> pretations. In making this decision, the jury is not likely to favor
> the opinion of the experts produced by the employer.
>   (2) The desirability of making various dust diseases compensable
> under properly drawn workmen's compensation laws. One of the
> speakers stated that "the strongest bulwark against future disaster
> for industry is the enactment of properly drawn occupational
> disease legislation." Such legislation would (a) eliminate the jury
> and empower a Medical Board to pass upon the existence of the
> disease and the extent of the disability; (b) eliminate the shyster
> lawyer and the quack doctor since fees would be strictly limited
> by the law …

The group decided to set up a committee to compile a database
of information on industrial dust problems and to push for the
workers' compensation laws. Under the auspices of the Mellon Institute, they collected $25,000 in $500 pledges from each company
and got to work. The resulting consortium was described by one
attorney: "Although the Air Hygiene Foundation is approaching
various problems relating to air hygiene from an unbiased viewpoint, it is, nevertheless, the creature of industry and is the one
institution upon which employers can rely completely for a sympathetic appreciation of their viewpoint."

Two years later, the group obtained part of what it was looking
for: a set of health-based standards upon which it could rely as a

defense against asbestosis claims. In 1938 the U.S. Public Health Service and Metropolitan Life insurance company teamed up to produce a study conducted by former surgeon general Waldemar C. Dreessen, who compiled health data and dust exposure levels for 541 textile workers at four plants in North Carolina. The circumstances were not ideal: the workers were young and therefore hadn't much chance to get sick yet; fiber counts could only be estimated and were low for that time period—consistently under 12 fibers per millimeter of air. It proved impossible for Dreessen to project from these factors the incidence of disease over a lifetime of working with asbestos and the effects of much higher fiber counts in places like Libby. Nonetheless, Dreessen hesitantly concluded, "It would seem that if the dust concentration in asbestos factories could be kept below five million particles, new cases probably would not appear."

Dreessen was wrong, of course, but his numbers stood for more than three decades as a self-inflicted guideline that industries were happy to adopt. Such a rule offered stability and legal protection. The standard didn't have to be safe or healthy, so long as it was perceived as such. And as the story of the Saranac Laboratory shows, it was perception, not health, in which the industry primarily was interested.

Among the many industrial groups formed in the 1930s and 1940s to deal with asbestos problems was the Industrial Hygiene Foundation. The foundation counted among its members the corporate giants of the day—Johns-Manville, Raybestos Manhattan, and Owen-Corning Fiberglass—but future Grace subsidiary Davison Chemical belonged as well. The foundation funded research, and one of its main beneficiaries was the Saranac Laboratory.

Saranac was the research facility of the Trudeau Institute, a sanatorium dedicated to the study and treatment of tuberculosis. Located on the picturesque Saranac Lake in New York, the laboratory was hired by the Industrial Hygiene Foundation to come up with hard data on the health effects of asbestos exposure. In doing so, the foundation acquired the services of the man who would make the first irrefutable link between asbestos and cancer two decades before the independent medical community could conclu-sively make that connection: Dr. Le Roy Gardner.

Gardner worked so closely with his patrons, he considered him-self an insider. In a 1946 letter to Johns-Manville, he wrote, "It is to collect and publish more reliable information on this [the asbestos-cancer link] and other little appreciated phases of the asbestos problem that I hope we may have the opportunity to review all films of Johns-Manville employees. Somebody should do this for the asbestos industry in the United States. I believe that 'some-body' should be outside of the industry, as obviously it would carry more weight. I hope, before I die, the opportunity may be afforded us." The statement was prophetic—Gardner died in November of that year, and it took until 1995 for his groundbreaking research to get published, long after the independent medical community had caught up with the secret corporate data.

The most complete account of Gardner's asbestos research at Saranac and the subsequent censorship of his findings is an article by Dr. Gerrit Schepers, himself a former director at Saranac. Schepers, in an article entitled "Chronology of Asbestos Cancer Discoveries: Experimental Studies of the Saranac Laboratory" pub-lished in the 1995 *American Journal of Industrial Medicine*, asserted that there is no question Gardner found cancer in mice exposed to chrysotile asbestos fibers in a 1942 study, and that this information was subsequently suppressed by his successor after Gardner died in 1946. The first part of his analysis Schepers based on Gardner's handwritten lab notes, the second on his personal experience at the lab beginning in 1949.

As early as 1930, Schepers wrote, Dr. Gardner observed unusual reactions to chrysotile asbestos in the lungs of mice. "Dr. Gardner did not publish these research findings in technical journals," Schepers explained, "for his work was performed on behalf of in-dustrial sponsors, from whom he did not have permission to pub-lish." Next, Gardner proposed a study "to test the carcinogenicity of lifetime inhalation of long fiber chrysotile dust on cancer resis-tant mice." When Schepers came on the scene in 1949, he asked Gardner's successor, Dr. Arthur Vorwald, about the proposal and was left with the impression that the study was never conducted. "I asked Vorwald what cancer research was conducted at the Laboratory on chrysotile asbestos. He said none had been attempted, none was contemplated, and none was needed, for in his opinion pneumoconiosis did not cause cancer. ..."

Among Schepers's duties at the lab was to look into the asbestos-cancer link. He was on assignment from the Pneumoconiosis Bureau of the South African government, which was at that time considering asbestos-related cancer as a compensable occupational disease. So he began to dig into Gardner's files, and eventually came across a set of mouse slides, some of them showing "malignant neoplasms," or malignant tumors. "These mice had been exposed to chrysotile fibers, but showed no asbestosis, just cancers. I also found nine human lung cancer and two mesothelioma cases in a file identified as 'Quebec Asbestos Workers.' Dr. Vorwald gave no explanation."

The results of Gardner's work appeared to be that he found "81.8% cancers in mice exposed to chrysotile dust." Schepers took this information, as well as the human cancer cases, to the Quebec Asbestos Mining Association, among others. "When I returned to the Saranac Laboratory about a month later after consulting with officials of Canadian industries, university medical schools, and government departments, Dr. Vorwald took me to task for mentioning the Laboratory cancer data. ... I also found that all the cancerous mouse slides had been lifted from the files. Dr. Vorwald said that Lanza, Smith, Cartier, and Sabourin all had honed in on him immediately after my visit to Canada. Dr. Vorwald said that he was reprimanded for being derelict in letting me, 'a foreigner,' see the patently sensitive data on chrysotile carcinogenicity, without being warned not to talk about what I had observed."

Lanza is Dr. Anthony Lanza, a man who wore multiple hats in the greater asbestos drama. Lanza was director of the Institute of Industrial Medicine at New York University, where Schepers was a graduate student. He was assistant medical director at the Metropolitan Life insurance company. Plus he was a research physician who conducted his own study of asbestos workers from 1929 to

1931. In this capacity, Lanza changed his data at the request of Johns-Manville attorney Vandiver Brown to downplay the danger of asbestos, including the fact that more than half of his study cohort—67 of 126—were suffering from asbestosis.

"Next Dr. Lanza took me to Mr. Vandiver Brown, the chief attorney for Johns-Manville and also the asbestos consortium which had sponsored Gardner's asbestos research up to the point where he mentioned cancer. Mr. Brown had the original of my university thesis, which doubled as my report to the South African Government. Brown asked me to withdraw this. I told him I could not and that I already had mailed my report to Johannesburg. Mr. Brown flew immediately to South Africa to retrieve my report from the Department of Mines officials. This merely heightened their interest in what I had to say."

Meanwhile, in what Schepers interpreted as a preemptive move, the Johns-Manville medical director published a report on the Quebec asbestos workers, mentioning the Saranac cancer cases in passing. And Vorwald published in 1951 what was purported to be a synopsis of Gardner's work. "Gardner's descriptions were copied across almost verbatim," Schepers wrote, "except that the mouse data are not mentioned."

In 1953, Schepers succeeded Vorwald as director of Saranac, and wrote that over the next decades he encouraged everyone involved—who were not otherwise bound by contract to keep their research private—to publish on the asbestos-cancer link. No one did, and Vorwald died in 1976. "Did Dr. Vorwald discover that chrysotile caused lung cancer? He most assuredly did, both in mice and men. The fact that he never published anything on such an important matter may be a mystery, but not if one considers that for almost three decades he had served as a defense litigation expert for the asbestos industries. It would hardly have been of value to his sponsors to permit release in scientific publications of the very incriminating data he commanded."

More than two decades after the asbestos industry researchers made the cancer connection, an independent doctor working at Mt. Sinai Hospital in New York released the results of his research in a series of articles that made the name Selikoff synonymous with asbestos. In 1964, Dr. Irving Selikoff laid to rest any doubts about the cancer link with a study finding cancer deaths among asbestos insulation workers at more than seven times the normal rate. Even more shocking was his 1968 report in which he described the synergistic effect between smoking and asbestos exposure, finding the risk level for cancer at ninety-two times the rate for the nonsmoking, non-asbestos-exposed population. He pushed these details at medical conferences and in the popular press, to the consternation of asbestos companies. "Dr. Selikoff started to speak out publicly to our knowledge in early 1969 around New York and, in fact, got the fireproofing sub-contractors and sprayed fiber manufacturers association to form a committee to set standards to improve job conditions," Grace executive Thomas Egan wrote in 1970. "The general feeling was that he would go away if he was treated gently. But this was not to be, as he stepped up his attack. ..." Testifying before a congressional subcommittee in 1973, Selikoff predicted that if America didn't change its ways, one million workers would die of asbestos-related diseases by the turn of the century.

By the late 1960s, Selikoff's studies and the resulting publicity were having their intended effects. Cities and states began regulating asbestos use: New York, Chicago, Boston, California. Federal agencies followed suit. The Bureau of Mines, Occupational Safety and Health Administration, Environmental Protection Agency, National Institute of Occupational Safety and Health, and Consumer Products Safety Council (CPSC) all regulated their corner of the asbestos market. Legal workplace exposure limits fell steadily as a waterfall through the 1970s, from 12 fibers/ml to 5, to 2, and finally to OSHA's current limit of .1 fibers/ml of air. The CPSC banned a few products in the late 1970s—fake fireplace logs and asbestos hair-dryers. Then in the 1980s, the EPA waged a widely publicized campaign to remove asbestos from school buildings.

But it was one of the first asbestos rules that was the most far-reaching and that gave Grace fits over one of its most popular products, Monokote. In 1973 the EPA won authority under the federal National Emission Standard for Asbestos law to ban friable (or easily crumbled), spray-on "asbestos-containing materials" with greater than 1 percent asbestos content by dry weight—a category that included Grace's Monokote-3. The recipe for Monokote-3 called for about 12 percent commercial chrysotile asbestos added to a blend of nearly 30 percent of Libby's vermiculite grade 3, and rounded out with 58 percent gypsum.

Companies got around the requirement to some extent because of the word "friable." Theoretically, asbestos that was bound up in some way in a material that wouldn't crumble and disperse the fibers was safer. It became common for insulation and fireproofing manufacturers to "bind" their fibers with organic material like cellulose and rock wool. And there was good reason to do so. In the era of skyscrapers, spray-on insulation was in great demand. The construction industry found value in fireproofing that flowed easily through hoses and could be pumped to great heights. In the case of the World Trade Center, according to Project Engineer Hyman Brown, Grace's Monokote was the fireproofing of choice, making it possible to use lightweight beams that otherwise might melt too quickly in case of fire. "Theoretically you have fireproofing on a beam to retard the melting of the steel," he says, "and you put the fireproofing on the beam with the theory that the fire will only burn at about 1,200 degrees Fahrenheit, and therefore the fireproofing will do its job." The engineers did not anticipate a fire fed by jet fuel, which simply burned too hot for the fireproofing to handle, Brown says.

Grace president Bill Corcoran told reporters in the aftermath of the towers' collapse that his company's products were not used in the World Trade Center's construction. But Allen Morrison, spokesperson for the Port Authority of New York and New Jersey (which owned the towers), contradicts Corcoran, saying that Grace's product was used to fireproof the buildings, though he could not give any details as to the quantity used.

By the time construction on the World Trade Center's steel structure began in 1968, the buzz over asbestos disease began to crescendo. Grace won the contract to supply fireproofing for the project, but was savvy enough not to refer to its product as Monokote. "In an effort to provide the proper fire protection and provide heat flow into the column it was felt that a dense vermiculite-gypsum plaster could best fulfill the needs," reads an April 1968 analysis prepared by Grace, titled "Study of the Interior Fire Protection Requirements of the Exterior Columns for the World Trade Center Project." EPA toxicologist Chris Weis says this "dense vermiculite-gypsum plaster" was likely Monokote-3. "They were calling it whatever they had to call it to market it," he says. "The vermiculite imparted the fireproofing. Unfortunately, it may have been, you know, 5 to 15 percent tremolite asbestos."

In 1970, the public outcry caught up with Grace. That April, the City of New York enacted a series of restrictions on sprayed asbestos-containing materials that effectively prohibited the company's work at the World Trade Center. According to an article in the May 7 *Engineering News-Record*, "Sprayed-asbestos fireproofing operations on steel-framed buildings halted last week in New York City. The stoppage resulted from regulations written after medical research showed that asbestos fibers can cause cancer of the pulmonary and gastro-intestinal tracts if ingested." The stoppage affected four buildings in New York, according to the article. "Ironically, the World Trade Center project was the first and only building in the city where the spray contractor had taken precautions to prevent scattering of dried asbestos. ... The job, however, lacked the vacuum cleaning operation as required by the regulations." Workers had only insulated the first seventy floors of the North Tower at that point, according to a subsequent story in the *Newark Evening News*. But as one internal corporate memo implies, Grace had anticipated such a move at least since 1969. "We should do everything we can to speed up our search for a substitute for the asbestos in our Monokote," District Manager Jim Cintani wrote on October 3, 1969. "We would certainly be at a distinct advantage if we could say our product did not contain any asbestos." By the time Grace was kicked off the job in 1970, it had a substitute product to offer. "We are currently working on modifying the Mono-Kote formula to replace the asbestos and have fire tests scheduled with the Underwriters' Laboratories in the next two months," Grace official Rod Vining wrote on April 10, 1970, three days before New York City's new regulations took effect. "We are currently working on trying to get a switch made at the World Trade Center and other building projects."

Grace won approval from the City of New York in 1971 to use its new product, Monokote-4, which the company marketed as being a "non-asbestos-fireproofing product." And truly, the company figured out a way to substitute a cellulose-based fiber for the 12 percent commercial chrysotile in Monokote-3, but still used Libby vermiculite grade 3. And that ore, Weis says, was the baddest of the bad. "Size 3 probably had more tremolite asbestos than any of the Libby ore," he says.

According to engineer Brown, now a professor at the University of Colorado in Boulder, that switch was made at the World Trade Center. "So I can tell you right now that [Monokote-3] was used in the first building, most of the first building, and [Monokote-4] was used for the rest of the first building and the second building because we were told that [Monokote-4] did not have asbestos in it."

Two hundred forty-four steel beams ringed each of the towers, with more beams around each elevator core, and steel trusses supporting every one of 110 floors in both buildings. Though Brown doesn't recall specifically how much Monokote went into the towers, a 1970 news report said the project called for an estimated 5,000 tons of sprayed fireproofing. If the contractors used only Monokote, following Weis's calculations that adds up to somewhere between 250 and 750 tons of tremolite asbestos.

AS MORE LOCAL AND FEDERAL regulations closed in on Grace in the early 1970s, the company scrambled to protect itself. In San Francisco and Canada, company managers used the time-honored strategy of doing their dirtiest work at night to avoid trouble. On August 6, 1971, a Zonolite executive from the Bay Area said that he expected problems from local inspectors. "Dear Fred," he wrote to Grace official Fred Eaton. "A call from Aase today. Wanted to know how much of our total production was #4. Naturally, I got nervous. I told him offhand I'd guess at 25% to 30%. He said you had stated that it was about 40%. Told him you could be right but that I'd have to check the records to be sure. He said that wasn't necessary that with that much of our total in #4 the area inspector would have to have been by here when we were running it. ...

"We'll be careful about keeping the cyclones clean and getting out as much #4 at night as we can. I think our 'friendly neighborhood inspector' will be by frequently for the next few weeks."

In a similar situation three months later in Winnipeg, Manitoba, Grace officials discussed complaints the city had passed along regarding Zonolite's emissions. "We had been aware for some time that the residents in the area have been complaining when we have been making Masonry Fill. For this reason most of the Masonry Fill has been made on the night shift when no one can see the emission."

The EPA's new rules effectively banning Monokote-3 nationwide were set to go into effect in July 1973. Grace prepared for this by instructing its salespeople to dump as much Monokote-3 on the market as possible. "All stocks of MK-3 should be used prior to July 4, 1973. Please arrange to have any warehouse stocks shipped to one of your customers in time for use of this material prior to the above date," wrote Zonolite district manager William Culver on May 24, 1973. "We will be unable to accept any MK-3 for return or credit."

Grace had labeling problems as well: inspectors upbraided the company and its wholesale customers for mislabeling or failing to label bags of Monokote in Florida, Texas, and Minnesota. When Washington state inspectors called Grace on the carpet in December 1973 for a similar violation, the company sent its top toxicologist and foot soldier, Harry Eschenbach, to smooth things over. According to a state memo summarizing this conference, Eschenbach defended the integrity of the corporation by blaming local managers: "This product was supposed to have been eliminated from their line, however, sales and the local plant accepted the order to match the material for the Spokane Airport expansion program without the knowledge of the corporate office. ... The application of Zonolite for insulating purposes may not pose a health

[sic] with respect to asbestos fibers. Zonolite itself does not have asbestos added as did the acoustical plastic."

As the decade advanced, the existence of asbestos in Monokote-4 became a closely guarded secret. The issue came to the fore of company policy in 1977, when Grace held a meeting at headquarters in Cambridge. In a confidential memo convening the group, Grace official Chip Wood directed that "customer, user or government inquiries with respect to tremolite in our plants, products, or use environments will receive straightforward and candid responses with respect to the data and measurements which we have gathered and which are relevant to their respective situations." A few days later, the company clarified this policy of honesty: "Detailed product formulation information is not divulged to any outside individual or organization without approval by Division Management and on a case by case basis. ... The respirable tremolite content is so small as to be considered de minimus, i.e., trifling and insignificant. Therefore, the fact that minute amounts of tremolite may be present is detailed product formulation information. Accordingly, all communications to outsiders involving questions of 'asbestos content' in the subject [of] mixed products will be dealt with as follows: 'There is no asbestos in _____.'"

Two months later, Wood elaborated further: "In the case of mixed products (MONOKOTE and soil mixes), tremolite is detectable only through the use of internally developed analytical procedures which require elaborate techniques not commonly recognized or employed in the scientific community for detection of asbestos. For this reason, we are taking the position with all but authorized government authorities that our mixed products are 'non-asbestos' products."

With this new Monokote, Grace filled a void left when other insulation manufacturers were forced out of the market because of the EPA ban. "By 1977, Monokote was America's leading fireproofing material," the *New York Times* reported in 2001. "Grace estimates that it was used on 60 to 80 percent of the roughly 150,000 steel frame structures built during the 1970s and '80s." In its 1999 annual report, the company boasted, "Grace concrete admixtures, cement additives, masonry products, waterproofing, and fireproofing are hard at work in virtually every major construction project around the world. Grace products are integral to the World Trade Center in New York, the London Underground, the Bank of China Tower in Hong Kong, Berkeley Square in Glasgow, Scotland and the City Centre in Kuala Lumpur. ..."

WHO IS TO SAY THE GREED that bound asbestos to steel wouldn't inevitably find some release, reach across the decades, and inexorably attract a like evil to itself? And when it did, the problem was as vast and amorphous as the hatred that had unwittingly spawned it: What do you do with a swirling dust cloud probably containing hundreds of tons of asbestos, blowing with the wind in and out of densely populated neighborhoods? EPA director Christine Todd Whitman's initial response was to simply reassure people that they were safe.

"We are very encouraged that the results from our monitoring of air quality and drinking water conditions both in New York and near the Pentagon show that the public in these areas is not being exposed to excessive levels of asbestos or other harmful substances," Whitman announced in a September 18, 2001, press release. "Given the scope of the tragedy from last week, I am glad to reassure the people of New York and Washington, D.C. that their air is safe to breath [sic] and their water is safe to drink."

As the press repeated Whitman's words, the dust blanketed Lower Manhattan. EPA teams collected air samples around the clock at ten stations near Ground Zero, and later doubled the number of collection points. They analyzed the samples, posting data collated hourly on the Internet. The asbestos counts spiked and dropped with the breeze. Agency scientists took both air and bulk dust samples from inside a number of nearby buildings, including their own office, and analyzed the percentage of asbestos content. Rescue workers within a half block of the site, the press release stated, were given "appropriate protective equipment." The agency announced on September 14 that it "has initially budgeted $600,000 to provide technical assistance and response support.

More than 3,000 respirators, 60 self-contained breathing apparatus machines, and 10,000 specially-equipped protective suits are on the way to these disaster sites."

But because reliable eyewitnesses say many rescue workers were not wearing good respirators (or were not wearing respirators at all); because the EPA used top technology to analyze the asbestos in its own offices and a less accurate method for everyone else's air; because agency spokespeople misled the public about asbestos laws; because she did not take the lead in informing and protecting New Yorkers but initially left the staggering job of cleaning the building interiors up to the beleaguered city, Christine Todd Whitman is not this story's hero. Cate Jenkins is.

Jenkins, a senior chemist with the EPA's hazardous waste division, would hate that characterization, and would likely argue that it is not her courage that's important. It's the data. "Cate has done nothing but collect factual, empirical information, turn it into PDF files, and post it on the Web," EPA toxicologist Chris Weis explains to me from his office in Denver. "And what it's done is it's taken the public relations machine that the EPA had going after the collapse and basically turned it on its ear. 'Cause what was being said, and what was being said to the press, was not consistent with the hard facts, the real data.

"What Cate did was nothing more than get the real data and go to the real regulations—including Libby information—and post that on the Web. ... It's incredibly interesting. There's a huge brouhaha in New York City and Washington about this."

When I ask Jenkins how she came to be the one collecting all this information—hinting that she must have landed in some hot water—she cuts me short, saying that even her refusal to talk about her motives is off the record. I am not to quote her. Jenkins's analysis, however, speaks for itself.

The EPA, she pointed out in one memo, detected asbestos at levels as high as 0.045 fibers/ml in the ambient air near Ground Zero in the weeks after the attack. This compares with an average of 0.009 fibers/ml in Libby homes where asbestos was detected. Cancer rates, she said, are generically calculated to increase by 4.8

people per 1,000 at asbestos levels of 0.019 fibers/ml. That figure is 4,750 times larger than the number that triggers EPA action; by law the agency is compelled to act whenever the excess cancer risk exceeds one in a million.

There were no perfectly tailored regulations for the agency to turn to at the scene of the World Trade Center disaster, so the EPA adapted a law it uses to protect children from asbestos in school buildings. "In evaluating data from the World Trade Center and the surrounding areas, EPA is using a protective standard under AHERA, the Asbestos Emergency Response Act, to evaluate the risk from asbestos in the outdoor and indoor air," one agency statement reads. "This is a very stringent standard that is used to determine whether children may re-enter a school building after asbestos has been removed or abated. ... To determine asbestos levels, air filters are collected from monitoring equipment through which air in the school building has passed and viewed through a microscope. The number of structures—material that has asbestos fibers on or in it— is then counted. The measurements must be 70 or fewer structures per square millimeter [s/mm^2] before children are allowed inside."

Seventy structures are equivalent to 0.01 fibers/ml. The EPA has taken to calling this the "school re-entry standard," and it sounds reassuring. The problem, Jenkins wrote, is that the 70 structures figure is obsolete, a construct to account for laboratory error. "Analysts have the choice of using either polycarbonate filters or methyl cellulose filters," she wrote. "Polycarbonate filters have asbestos fibers in the filter material itself. The AHERA clearance test was designed to allow for the presence of the asbestos in the polycarbonate filters, so it set the level at 70 s/mm^2 to allow for this contamination. Typically, the methyl cellulose filters are used today because it is understood that using polycarbonate filters would result in finding some asbestos as part of the lab background."

So what AHERA really calls for, Jenkins said, is a finding of zero asbestos fibers.

PIOTR CHMIELINSKI WAS AMONG THE many industrial hygienists called to action after the World Trade Center collapsed. A world-class kayaker who has traveled the Amazon River from its source in the Andes to its end in the Atlantic Ocean, Chmielinski was well into his second life as a family man and new career as co-founder of the HP Environmental company when the World Trade Center was bombed in 1993. He happened to be nearby, inspecting another building, and so was quickly on the scene and hired to screen the air quality in the wake of that attack. After the 2001 tragedy, authorities divided Ground Zero and the surrounding blocks into quadrants, and the construction company responsible for the northeast section hired Chmielinski's firm to do its sampling and testing. What Chmielinski and his partner, Hugh Granger, found shook the city like a second wave of attacks: despite the EPA's assurances to the contrary, there were high levels of asbestos in the air and dust.

To say "high levels of asbestos" is a little misleading, since *any* asbestos is considered by the government to be dangerous; consequently, *detectable* asbestos fibers are a big red flag of warning. Individual asbestos fibers are measured by the micron—an infinitesimal scale requiring specialized microscopes and sampling equipment. Scientists examine air and dust samples at magnifications of up to 20,000. But despite this exactitude, the microscopic world of an asbestos fiber is fraught with politics and controversy.

First, there's the tension between finding a safe level of exposure and one the industry finds to be practical. While asbestos is a carcinogen, and government health agencies across the board do their work on the premise that there is no safe level of exposure to a carcinogen, it's a controversy that has the EPA and federal Occupational Safety and Health Administration at odds.

Both of the laws used regularly by the EPA—the Asbestos Hazard Emergency Response Act and the Asbestos School Hazard Detection and Control Act—state that there is no safe level of exposure to asbestos, and mandate that public areas be made as clean as so-called background levels, which are generally higher in urban areas, lower in the countryside.

"Of course we don't know how to go below background in the outdoors unless we live in little shells that we walk around in," says

OSHA research scientist Dan Crane, who has been working with asbestos since he signed on with the agency in 1977. "There is a natural background of these fibers in the air. … In industry, technology is such that we'll control down to where we can, or where industry can get down to."

None of this, Crane warns, is considered safe.

"Asbestos is a known carcinogen, okay? There's a group of people who would argue that there's a safe level of asbestos. There's a group of people out there who say if you get below a certain level of asbestos, it's safe, there's no enhanced risk of asbestosis or mesothelioma or lung cancer or anything else. On the other hand, the most accepted paradigm is that there is no safe level. Zero is safe. All right? So you really and truly have two camps. The government, of course, is in the camp that has a real risk assessment that says we see no safe level. We'll have a permissible exposure level as low as we can feasibly measure it, as low as industry can feasibly control."

"Feasible," the EPA's Paul Peronard explains, doesn't just mean possible, but financially expedient. "The actual implementing law for OSHA has a second test for a rulemaking. One, they have to consider the health standard, and two, they have to consider the practicability of requiring an industry to meet the standard. So there's a means test to it. They have to say, 'Okay, how much would it cost to meet the standard?' And they actually compare that versus the incremental health benefits for lowering the standard further. They're required to do that by law. The other thing that the OSHA standard does is it assumes that you have a healthy adult, and that he or she is in a medical monitoring program getting regular checkups, and has protective gear available to them, so there are some other hygiene factors going on that will offer additional protection."

OSHA's limit, Peronard says, is not "appropriately protective for nonoccupational exposures. We typically look almost two orders of magnitude lower. …"

"So that would be like .001?" I ask.

"Yeah, and actually sometimes less than that depending on the fiber size distribution. The more longer, skinnier fibers you have, the lower that number goes. The 0.001 or thereabouts is something that we associate with about 1 in 1,000 cancer risks if it's a chrysotilic fiber. One of the problems is, our analytical capability is right at that detection level. We're having a hard time seeing levels lower than that, which is one of the reasons there's not an EPA risk number for asbestos for nonoccupational settings."

A second point of contention arises over analytical techniques. Some scientists—including those working for OSHA—use a method called phase contrast microscopy to measure the asbestos content of air samples. In Libby the EPA has relied on a technique called transmission electron microscopy (TEM) and its sister technology, scanning electron microscopy. A third method, polarized light microscopy, is used to measure the asbestos in bulk dust samples— to see whether a bag of Monokote, for instance, meets the EPA's limit of no more than 1 percent asbestos by dry weight. Under the right circumstances TEM can be far more accurate, but it is about ten times more expensive than phase contrast, and so industries prefer to use the latter. Also weighing in favor of phase contrast is the fact that it's the basis of the only model available that correlates exposure and disease.

OSHA research scientist Dan Crane says this cost-cutting is not necessarily a bad thing. "The transmission electron microscope sees many more fibers than does phase contrast," Crane says. "But in the phase contrast microscope you look at nearly a full square millimeter of material, and in the transmission electron microscope you look at less than 10 percent of that. And the fibers are distributed not uniformly on a filter; they're laid down at random. So there's higher incidence of error associated with the transmission electron microscope than there is with the phase contrast microscope. You're looking at a smaller piece of it. There's a higher chance that you find a high spot or a low spot. It doesn't correlate very well across the board.

"What you get, however, with the TEM is, you're able to tell what the minerals are that you're looking at generally, most of the time."

Scientists know they are missing a great number of fibers when they use phase contrast, Crane says, but the technique is good enough to use as an indicator of disease. The disease index based on Waldemar Dreessen's 1938 data was analyzed using the phase contrast method, and since the two methods don't correlate well, scientists would have to conduct an entirely new study to put together a new index based on the transmission electron method. That, Crane says, is not going to happen.

"I can't take a twenty-year-old worker, expose him at .05 fibers per cc for twenty years, come back when he's forty, and look at that cohort of people and see how many of them died," he says. "When we do [phase contrast], we have a real good solid idea in a given industry how sick people are going to get. And that's valuable. That's valuable because we can use that then to control in an industry. We can keep the numbers down so that we get fewer and fewer people sick."

Because the cost difference is prohibitive—about $15 for a reliable phase contrast sample versus $150 and up for TEM—Crane sees no reason for OSHA to switch. "The fibers that we see in phase contrast represent the tip of the iceberg. We know, and we have always known, that there are many more fibers in a sample that are not seen by our microscope, that are represented by what we do count.

"It doesn't matter much because we actually use that as an index of disease. It matters a lot in the EPA side of the equation when you're trying to be clean, because you're trying to make sure that that building is clean."

But in New York, clean was the goal. The agency wasn't dealing with a homogenous healthy working-age population, people employed in carefully controlled environments, exposed to asbestos for eight hours a day with protective clothing and respirators. There were children and people with compromised respiratory systems, who in moving back to their apartments would be exposed for up to twenty-four hours a day, who in going back to their office jobs would put on a coat and tie, not a "self-contained breathing apparatus." In their hurry to reassure the public, the EPA used the less sensitive phase contrast, misrepresented the implications of their findings by calling the 70-structures formula "safe," and then to top it all off, sampled their own building using TEM. Most of the samples collected at the EPA building from September 13 through 17 tested negative. But not all. "On 14 September 2001, two dust samples were collected outside the building entrance, and three samples were collected inside the lobby. The initial TEM qualitative analysis did find chrysotile asbestos to be present in the dust at all locations, inside and outside the building," according to an EPA report excerpted by Jenkins. The EPA subsequently performed an asbestos abatement in its own office.

In a letter to New York Representative Jerry Nadler, Christine Todd Whitman defended this decision, saying, "EPA did not set a more stringent standard of cleanup for these federal buildings, and the lobby cleanup was consistent with the New York Department of Health advisory. After noting significant amounts of dust tracked into 290 Broadway and 26 Federal Plaza by workers responding at the World Trade Center, the General Services Administration asked EPA to clean the lobbies."

Piotr Chmielinski and Hugh Granger, too, chose to use TEM to analyze their section of the World Trade Center disaster site. "Transmission electron microscopy—there is no comparison," Chmielinski says, explaining this decision with a heavy Polish accent. "It is easier to spot smaller fibers a lot less in diameter and will pick up real fibers; that means it will not really look at the fibers which are cellulose or rock or any other components, any other fibers, but can detect asbestos type of forms. Instead of phase contrast microscopy, which you look at any fibers, asbestos fibers or cellulose fibers, it looks the same."

Chmielinski and Granger released their findings in an October 2, 2001, report that was posted briefly on the American Industrial Hygiene Association's website, but it was removed almost immediately. The plain numbers tell the story. The results of 11 ambient air samples taken from inside two buildings near the disaster site ranged from 0.008 fibers/ml to 5.36 fibers/ml, as detected by TEM. These same samples measured by phase contrast yielded nowhere near the same fiber counts—from less than 0.005 fibers/ml to a high of only 0.536 fibers/ml. When Chmielinski and Granger looked for

asbestos in the dust that had settled on surface areas in their quad-
rant northeast of the World Trade Center, and specifically north of
Building 7 from the WTC complex, their results ranged from 0.25
to as high as 0.75 percent. They also found asbestos fibers both with
and without the binders used to keep the fibers from becoming airborne. This means, Chmielinski says, that the binders failed. "Normally, it's a natural binder which holds those bundles of fibers
together or was artificial binder which is applied like in the floor
tiles or adhesives," he says. "And all that was crumbled to pieces
and individual fibers were released and being independent."

Although the asbestos content Chmielinski and Granger found
in their bulk dust samples was within the EPA's 1973 standard allowing up to 1 percent asbestos in spray-on materials, that doesn't
mean it is safe. That standard was tailored to a specific set of circumstances: a construction zone or the like, involving tents and
proper breathing equipment, protective clothing, and with the so-
called asbestos-containing material wetted down. According to
Chmielinski and Granger's report, "the particle size of the surface
residue is very fine (and dry), a condition not typically encountered during routine asbestos removal projects. … There is every
indication, and it is reasonable to assume, that under commonly
encountered conditions the components of the fine surface residue
will become airborne and thus available for inhalation by workers.
Under conditions where rapid dilution of the air does not occur,
such as within building structures, it should be anticipated that
very small asbestos fibers may become airborne and remain in the
breathing zone of workers for extended periods."

The key phrase in that paragraph is "very small asbestos fibers."
It is another factor that accounts for some of the discrepancy between the EPA's and Chmielinski's numbers. The EPA counts only
fibers of a certain size: they must be at least 5 microns in length,
with an "aspect ratio" (length to width) of at least three to one.
"These are the fibers that are small enough to be inhaled deeply
into the lungs ('respirable size'), but also large enough to be retained by the lungs," EPA whistleblower Cate Jenkins explained.
But at the World Trade Center, everything was pulverized.

"Some people will say it doesn't matter what size of fibers; they are dangerous to the human health," Chmielinski says. "Another group will say, 'No, fibers smaller than some size will not affect you.' At that point here, at the World Trade Center, the issue was not only how small but how many of them. This is an issue, but really at that point we didn't want to comment previously, and I will not like to comment what I think myself. The only one statement I will say, if you have too many of something, even water or good meal, it can affect you and we have the same issue here."

What Chmielinski also will say is that these tiny, pulverized fibers are more likely to stay airborne. "Because it's very small, it's a lot easier to become airborne. And if there are fibers, small asbestos fibers in the air, they will stay in the air a lot longer, and they are a lot more difficult to be cleaned, released, taken away. If your sofa's affected, very difficult to get those fibers out because they went far deep to the surface of that type of covering.

"And now, as an example of the explanation of why we've got a problem there, normally asbestos fibers is like a bundle. That one bundle—it was broken to pieces out of one fiber—now becomes hundreds or even thousands of small teeny, tiny fibers. Definitely those smaller fibers will stay and will be suspended in air a lot longer than the bigger fiber, which will stay in the air for some time but will fall easier down to the surface."

National Geographic Adventure magazine editor Mark Jannot followed Chmielinski around Ground Zero on October 2, 2001, the day Chmielinski and Granger released their report detailing their findings. More graphic than the numbers they reported was the scene Mark Jannot described in the February 2002 issue of his magazine: "Cutting diagonally across from the south west corner of the Site, we enter One World Financial Center, flashing our passes to the chubby, baby-faced security guard sitting in the lower-level loading dock. The guard is wearing no protective gear, and he nervously asks about the air. Chmielinski answers without hesitation. 'If you are working in this building eight hours a day,' he says, 'you should be wearing your respirator.'"

When they encounter another guard wearing a "flimsy rubber-band-and-toilet-paper particulate" mask, Chmielinski warns the man it is not sufficient protection against asbestos fibers. "'You scared those guys to death,'" Jannot said he remarked to Chmielinski. "'Better I tell them now than have them hear it in two, three months. Think what that does to their mind then.'"

That scene, Chmielinski tells me, was not uncommon. "Well, people were not informed. In those days, people were concerned about finding the life, people who were alive. And there was not so much concern about your own life or your companion's life. At this point, even firemen and policemen, they looked really silly if they were wearing those respirators because they were looking for their companions in the debris."

As for the censorship of their report, Chmielinski says that while they were told it was taken off the Web by accident because of a computer glitch, it was never posted again. But that, he says, is not important. Word got out and people began to be more careful about their own health. And eight months after the disaster, the EPA announced it would lead the effort to clean out people's apartments after all.

Forty years from now, the fuss may turn out to have been unwarranted. Or Selikoff's warnings may have played out accurately, though in a scenario he could never have predicted. One thing is for certain: if New Yorkers become ill with asbestosis, they will find, as Libby's victims have, that there are few places to turn for justice. On April 2, 2001, W.R. Grace became one of the last of the asbestos giants to file for bankruptcy.

The Fisherman

The Libby dam lies about a dozen miles upstream from the Rainy Creek Road turnoff to Grace's old mine, but men who built the dam will tell you they often saw a huge cloud of dust rising from the mountain. "I'm one of them," says Royce Ryan, who moved to Libby in 1966 from Washington State to work as a supervisor on the dam project. "Just kind of a gray-white plume came up. And you could hear the rumble."

The cloud moved with the wind—some days toward town, some days north toward the construction workers. It doesn't much matter to Ryan now whether he was dosed with asbestos at the dam or later when he went to work for Grace dismantling the old dry mill. The end result is the same: he's nearly broke, two of his six children are sick with asbestosis, and his own health will only decline.

Ryan's run of bad luck started with one bad step in 1980 and hasn't ended yet. "It was the first snowfall. I got on the bus, work bus, went up to the mine. I was the first one to step off. ... The step was froze and I stepped on it, and my feet went out from underneath me and I landed on the steel edge on my lower back. I worked almost two years with it like that. I couldn't hardly get out of bed in the mornings." Three back surgeries later, Ryan was ready to go to work again, but Grace had no "limited duty" jobs at the mine or mill. After casting about for something he could do, Ryan finally gave up and went on Social Security. "And then I had a heart attack, stress, after that. And one thing led to another. I was immobile for almost eighteen months. Then I had to have open-heart surgery. I guess the cholesterol built up in my system so much from being immobile," he says. It was a tough time for Ryan, an avid outdoorsman. Camping and fishing, he says, are his life. He has spent countless hours on the Kootenai River, and one of his dreams is to go angling in south-central Montana, on the Big Hole and Madison Rivers. Right now, he says, he just doesn't have the money. His savings were used up by his health problems.

"It was about three years, seemed like my whole world come crashing down around me. A lot of stress. I applied for different jobs: wouldn't be accepted with my medical history. And then in 1981, when Ronald Reagan took office, when they cut all of the Social Security to disabled people, I was one of them. I had to prove that I was disabled. Went through thirteen, fourteen months. I finally ended up driving a school bus.

"Finally I got to court with Social Security in Kalispell here, and the judge ruled in my favor. Then I got my butt chewed out by him. He said, 'How could you—knowing that you had a heart attack and all these medical things wrong with you—drive a school bus, put those children at risk?' I told him I had to feed my family. And he gave me my Social Security back. Then I applied for my retirement and found out that I didn't have enough time in. I lacked three months of invested time and lost that battle in court too. So we've been living on Social Security ever since."

Ryan says he loved Libby and would have stayed there forever, but in the end simply couldn't afford it. "I had to sell everything we had. Live off it. We're at the last of it right now. All of our savings is gone. Medical." He and his wife moved to Kalispell in 1984 to be closer to the medical care he needed. And in 1998, a former coworker mentioned that he had heard they'd all been exposed to asbestos at the mine. Ryan went to a doctor who found asbestos tracks on his lungs, a diagnosis confirmed by Dr. Whitehouse in Spokane. He immediately lodged a lawsuit against Grace, but had his hearing postponed twice before the corporation filed for bankruptcy in 2001. "They did give me a very measly offer, and I wouldn't accept it," he says. "It would be equal to a month's pay, I'll tell you that." Ryan has since been chosen to represent Libby in bankruptcy court by serving on the personal injury committee.

In a move to save the bulk of its money from asbestos lawsuits, Grace spun off one of its most profitable subsidiaries in 1997 for $5 billion, leaving what will probably amount to a pittance for its asbestos victims in Montana as well as for its other creditors. "This was a great chance to split the packaging company away from the asbestos liabilities holding down our stock multiple," Grace chairman Albert Costello told the *New York Times* when the deal was announced.

So far, the effects of asbestosis have been minor compared with Ryan's other health problems. "The medication that the doctors prescribed for me was aggravating my blood pressure and a few other things," he says. "I just quit taking it." Ryan has no health insurance, only the coverage that Grace is providing to its Libby victims while the bankruptcy proceeds.

The year his corporation declared itself broke, Grace CEO Paul Norris made just over $3.4 million.

EIGHT

A Daughter's Revenge

THE QUESTION WAS PUT TO Gayla rather prophetically, and she was wise to take it seriously. "If I release the story, things are going to change forever." The Seattle reporter who broke the Libby story was asking her, What did she want to do? She hesitated to answer. "We were always afraid of ruining the jury pool in Libby," she explains.

It was only by chance that Libby victims could go to court at all: Montana's 1959 workers' compensation law funnels occupational claims through a separate adjudication process, which forbids workers from suing in civil court. The statute of limitations for filing a claim was set at three years. But within three years of what? Discovery of the illness? Death? The last day at work? When Louise Gidley, a miner's widow, approached Grace in 1982 about death benefits for her husband—a little more than a year after the Gidleys discovered he had lung cancer and two months after his death—the company argued that Jim Gidley had three years after his last day of employment in 1977 to file for workers' compensation. Mrs. Gidley was simply too late.

This time, however, even Grace's own managers balked at the orders sent down from Cambridge. "Jim was well known, well liked, and a model employee," manager Bill McCaig wrote to his bosses in 1983. "There is concern on the part of Earl Lovick and myself over the moral obligation involved when denial of benefits is based in failure to file a claim ... which would certainly have been approved at some point.

"We feel some settlement with Mrs. Gidley should be negotiated. Our image with our employees and with the community would suffer irreparable damage should this situation become public knowledge."

Grace, however, refused to take McCaig's advice and paid dearly for it. Louise Gidley sued the corporation, and when she won on appeal to the state supreme court, Grace lost the protection conferred by the 1959 law, which had until then kept employee health claims out of the court system. "Grace's defense was that 'oops, sorry, guys, but you have no claim under the occupational disease act, under the workers' comp act, because time has run,'" plaintiffs' attorney Roger Sullivan explains. "And of course we have immunity from suit under those acts so you can't sue us in court either.

"And so it was in the mid-1980s that the Montana Supreme Court said, 'No, that's wrong. You can't have it both ways.'"

From that day on, the cases started trickling in to local lawyers' offices. "What we started with was a small circle of men, old men, mine workers who had worked there a number of years ago," Sullivan recalls. "Then a concentric circle around that, if you can imagine, was the younger mine workers. Then the circles grew even further when we found out that family members, wives and unfortunately even children, were being diagnosed with asbestos-related disease. And then as the circle went out, we found that there were community members who had not even exposure from family members. Those were increasingly disturbing developments."

Sullivan's firm, headed by a Kalispell attorney named Dale McGarvey, handled—and settled—a number of Grace-related cases over the next decade. But until Gayla showed up with Les Skramstad in tow, McGarvey's lawyers had only pieces of the puzzle, enough to win settlements for each of the old miners. "They had snippets. They had enough information to get the money for the guys in the courts, and that was all they needed," Gayla says. "They had a few documents. Because they'd never followed up on a case after they settled, it was just 'Bring on the next one.'"

Gayla refused to be simply the next case in line, and it was through her acquaintance that the attorneys learned the difference between justice for one and justice for all.

"What happened then was that we were dealing with some extraordinary human beings who were concerned not only for the resolution of their own claims, but I think even more importantly to them, they were concerned for the future health of family members, community members," Sullivan explains. "And they weren't content just to let matters lie with the resolution of their claims. But if others were continuing to be exposed, then they wanted that matter resolved so that no one else would be hurt."

It was a happy accident that Benefield walked into the Kalispell law offices of McGarvey, Heberling and Sullivan: she chose them because they had listed a toll-free number in the yellow pages. At first they were skeptical about her chances of winning a wrongful death case in her mother's name. "I went to see [Roger Sullivan] and he said, 'I don't think so.' Then we got to talking."

It turned out they had an acquaintance in common: Gayla had once stolen a horse from one of Sullivan's clients. ("Actually it's a really funny story. I was drunk one night and stole Butch's horse from behind the Mint Bar. Twenty years ago, twenty-five years ago now. Last time I've been on a horse. It isn't the last time I was drunk, but it was the last time I drank and rode.") As they talked, Gayla told Sullivan about her friend, Les Skramstad. She'd recently run into Les at a Libby department store and knew he was doing poorly. "I said, 'Well, even if you can't do anything for me, here's my buddy Les.'"

With Les Skramstad's case, McGarvey's little law firm made history: in May 1997 they persuaded a jury to convict W.R. Grace for making Les sick and to award him $635,000—most of it punitive damages—for that. It was the first Libby case to go to a jury and one of the few guilty verdicts ever lodged against the multinational corporation. Even Jan Schlichtmann, the grandiose lawyer of *A Civil Action* fame, hadn't managed that feat. But the victory was bittersweet. The night before Les testified on his own behalf, he and Norita received a letter informing them that two of their kids—Laurel and Brent—had been diagnosed with asbestosis. "He was so angry that day," Gayla recalls. "He said, 'Those bastards.' Then he had to get up and testify and you could just see his anger up there." Adding insult to injury, Grace refused to pay Les what they owed him. Nearly a year later, the corporation offered him the $73,000 the jury had awarded simply for his medical bills and said, "Take it or leave it," threatening to delay payment further by appealing. By then his bills were mounting. Uninsured and desperate, Les took the money. "My life was bought pretty cheap," he admits.

But the diagnosis of two of Les and Norita's children was the first clue that Grace's dust was going to kill another generation.

REVENGE IS A TREACHEROUS DISH. The first bite may taste sweet, a fulfillment of one's dearest-held wishes. But no matter how justified, it can turn so slowly in your gut that you don't even notice the bitterness at the back of your throat until your body is wracked with the sickness of it. You've won your dream but paid for it with your soul. After their mother died, Gayla Benefield and Eva Thomson filed a wrongful-death lawsuit against Grace. At first no one believed Gayla when she insisted the case was not about money, that it was an apology she was after and, barring that, a guilty verdict against the W.R. Grace corporation. Benefield was pursuing Grace for the sheer satisfaction of it. As time progressed, Eva began to fear the effects revenge would take on her sister's spirit. She encouraged Gayla to settle out of court.

"I thought Gayla's anger was too great," she says. "We all thought if Gayla got it done with and behind her, she would be better for it." But Gayla refused to take the settlement talks seriously, even as she placated those around her by listening to Grace's offers. "We first went into settlement hearings, it was 'You don't have a case. We'll give you $10,000.'

"'Well,' I said, 'I don't want it.'

"'Yeah, but you don't have a case.'

"Well they got up to $35,000 that day. I said, 'Listen, if I don't have a case, why do you keep jumping it up by $10,000?'"

Gayla says she had watched her neighbors and friends settle for peanuts: $35,000 for Helen Bundrock, $400,000 for a supervisor's wife. There was, she says, neither rhyme nor reason to the amounts. In addition, the lawyers encouraged a culture of silence that further victimized the sick. It all came to a climax, she says, during the deposition phase of her trial when Dr. Richard Irons, the mountain climber who had tried to expose Grace in the 1970s, flew in to testify.

"The oddity is that when all these trials were going on, because Irons was going to testify or give a deposition, I couldn't communicate with him. These were Roger's rules. Roger was really paranoid: 'Grace is just gonna . . .'

"I said, 'So let 'em. What are they going to do?'"

She began to find out when Grace started deposing her daughters. "They deposed Jenny. I'm sure it was Jenny—I've got it right here. It is just disgusting. And they had Stacey crying during her deposition. They had my other friend madder than hell. Because they wanted to know why I was doing this, where my computer was, if I was doing all this over the computer, where the exact location of the computer. They acted like they were going to come in and confiscate the computer."

In another case they badgered a woman who was trying to obtain compensation for her husband's death: "'How do you know Gayla Benefield? When did you last meet with Gayla Benefield? How long did you talk to Gayla Benefield?' Like I was on trial, had nothing to do with the man who had died. They were trying me.

"I bowed my neck and thought, 'You're not pushing me around.' I watched them push so many people around. It was so pathetic to see these people go in, and they'd sign up at the law firms, and before they signed up they weren't allowed to talk to each other. Roger tried it on us. 'Don't talk to anybody, don't discuss your case with anybody, don't say anything at all. You get that money, don't talk about anything, just go die.' It was tragic. Roger and them had the goddamn gall to pull it. And they asked Les not to talk. It was me, Butch, and Les, all three of us.

"This was long before we broke the story, they said, 'Don't discuss it with each other.' And Les said, 'Hey, I'm sorry.' He says, 'If that's the way it's gonna be, forget it. I ain't going to trial. Nobody's gonna shut me up.'"

Gayla saw it as her duty to use her health to fight. "You wouldn't believe how many, over the years that I had gotten to know, had gone through the system and gotten their settlement and then called me so apologetic and said, 'Gayla, I'm sorry. I caved. I just couldn't make it into court.' And oh God, I can't even imagine. And I told 'em, I said, 'You know, save it for somebody who's healthy. Save it for a wrongful death or something.'

"It was a good feeling to say 'Get on with your life. Don't worry, somebody else will go to court. Somebody will get 'em.' 'Cause we always thought that first one to go to court, get that guilty verdict, God, it'd be across newspapers in the country. Boy," she says, laughing coarsely, "by the third one we knew it wasn't gonna happen."

Gayla and Eva's case came up on the court docket after Skramstad's. While Gayla was determined to put Grace on trial, the lawyers talked the sisters into going through the motions of settlement talks.

"Roger says you gotta put a dollar figure on it. Well, I said, '$100 billion.' Finally they decided $725,000. I said, 'That's ridiculous.' But we had to have a starting point. Well that day, W.R. Grace had come up to $75,000; my glorified attorneys on the other side had come down to $175,000. And you know, I said, 'This isn't right. You guys are coming down by the hundreds; they're coming up by the tens.'

"'Well that's the way we …'

"I said, 'Bullshit. Forget the money. Let's go to court.'"

"'No, we got to do this.'

"Finally, when that last thing went through, Roger and Allan were sitting right there. I said, 'I tell you what. Grace comes back and says we accept, the only way I'll take that check is over your left nut. So you better hope to chrissake they say no.' And they just looked at each other like 'Oh, fucked up this time.' I mean, my sister was sitting there just having a hissy-fit. But I just said, 'That's the only way I'll accept that check.'"

Fortunately for the men, Grace sat on their offer and the sisters' case went to trial. While Gayla was sure Eva's desire to settle was solely about greed, Eva says she was growing more and more concerned for her sister's mental health. The trial lasted two weeks. Roger had ordered the two women to sit with each other and be friendly about it, and on top of that, Gayla couldn't smoke in the courthouse. "I had to double-patch," she laughs, "practically was on Valium 'cause I had to sit next to her for two solid weeks. And so we sat together. We were just picture-perfect. Boy, the notes we were writing."

After each day in court, the settlement talks would resume. Grace kept upping the ante. First it was $500,000, then $600,000 and a letter of apology from the head of the company. "And I said, 'Well, that's getting close.' They thought money. I said, 'Can I publish this letter on the Internet?'

"'Absolutely not.'

"I said, 'What good would it do me?'

"'Well, you would have it, you would know.'

"I said, 'I know you killed my mother. I know you're never going to be sorry.' I said no."

She did, however, talk it over with her husband and kids first. "I called them all together and said they offered me half a million dollars to settle. And I said, 'Of course it'd be divided with Eva.' But I said, 'That's a lot of money. What do you think?' And every one of my kids didn't even bat an eye. They said, 'Mom, go for the guilty. It's just money.' And I thought, 'I raised these kids right.' Turned around to David. He says, 'Hey, I don't want to listen to you. Do what you want.' We're sitting there playing cribbage. I said, 'Do you realize I just turned down a half-million dollars?' He said, 'Yeah.' He says, 'I always knew you were nuts.'

"I mean, you know, *the money*. I could have done a lot of things with the money and helped the kids out.

"But the kids say, 'No, Mom. This is what everybody else has had to do.'"

After the jury heard the case and began considering a verdict, Grace offered Gayla and Eva $605,000, no letter, and a pledge to settle the case of one of Gayla's friends for $425,000. "That just put me around the bend. I sent back a message. I said, 'You bastards that's what's the matter with your company. I'm not sick, I'm not dying. You're giving me more money to shut up than my friend who's dying.'"

Even as the jury filed back in the courtroom, McGarvey asked Gayla if she was sure she didn't want the money. "Do you know I don't even remember anything? I thought all the lights were turned off in that courtroom. Because all I remember is just one person, a little spotlight shining on that person—it was really not. The verdict, and guilty. I don't remember what it was guilty for. That's all I remember that day."

The jury awarded Gayla and Eva $250,000 for their mother's wrongful death, but it was the verdict that started a settling in Gayla's heart. Her need for revenge, she says, was gone. "It wasn't vindictively done, but it was just a matter of the principle of the thing. It's all I ever learned about values. My father taught me to be honest, but by God, if you feel you're right, you stick to it. Don't you back down for anybody. And my mother was such a stickler on that—the principle, it was always the principle."

Gayla had fulfilled her mother's deathbed request, but she was pleased with the results far beyond what her mother had envisioned. "Just before Mom left for the care center, she grabbed my hand and she says, 'Gayla,' she says, 'You know my dying's going to make you and Eva rich.' ... She was thinking in terms of money because to her richness was money. And I'll tell you what, there's no amount of money in the world that could account for how rich her dying's made me feel. When I have somebody call me and say, 'Thank you, I made it through the system, I'm going to Arizona. I've only got a year or two, but we're just buying a motor home and getting the hell out of here.' ... Or like the woman who walked up to me in Rosauers the other day and she said, 'I just want you to know our family thinks you're just awesome.' I mean, that's the rich.

"People off the street will come up and say things like that. These old seniors will go, 'Way to go, Gayla!' And that's where the richness comes."

But there was darkness brewing yet in that moment of triumph. That Les and Norita's children were sick, that Helen Bundrock's young grandson—born in 1980 after Grace claimed it had cleaned up its act—had been diagnosed, coupled with the rumors of vermiculite in playgrounds and next to the Little League fields meant Libby was not a safe place to live. When Gayla's granddaughter Kate— Jen's middle girl—asked, "Am I going to die of it too, Grandma?"

it made her gut wrench. No one, *no one* should have to fear from childhood on that she will die as her mother did. In Gayla's heart, her grandchildren were everyone's grandchildren, and the job had fallen to her to save them all.

To be honest, prior to 1999, Libby did not want to be saved, and probably nobody knows that better than *Western News* editor Roger Morris. A Long Island native, Morris fell in love with the West while touring rural Colorado and Nebraska as a newspaper-man. He worked for papers in farm communities, ranch communities, tourist towns. He moved to Libby in July 1992, he says, and it was his first mining and logging town.

Soon after his arrival, he recalls having paid a visit to the county commissioners. "We were just talking," he says. "I asked them, I said, 'Is Grace leaving us any problems behind?' And they just about jumped down my throat.

"It was because they were losing a major employer. If you look back in the papers from '89 and '90, there were signs of this happening. And then when it was finally announced, the community formed committees and worked with the state and feds to try to keep Grace in operation. So they jumped down my throat and said, 'We solved all those problems and there's no problem and we're losing a great company, tax base'—the whole thing you hear from county commissioners, which they're paid to do. Okay. And I probably shouldn't have let it go then, but I didn't have any reason to believe it wasn't true. I wasn't hearing anything in the community at that time."

The idea that Morris's newspaper missed this story galls him. First of all, he points out, the *Western News* reported almost from day one in the 1920s that there was asbestos at the mine; it was just that no one knew how dangerous it was. By the 1960s, when Grace publicized a project to market its asbestos, no one batted an eye. But even under Morris's tenure the *Western News* covered the asbestos problem, albeit superficially. Six months or so before Morris arrived, the paper printed a story that explained the whole problem for everyone to read. "We printed a little story on an inside page about a filing, two filings on asbestos cases. It laid out everything. It was real brief. It was a 12-inch story across the top of the page. But everything was there that summarizes this whole problem. And I didn't hear anything about that." It was as if Libby operated in a vacuum: nothing got in or out. Only the miners' families cared much about their sick and dying men. Even in the year 2000 you could hear people say, "It's just a bunch of old miners." As if that were okay.

Through the 1990s, Morris trusted his reporters' judgment as they gave brief coverage to each of the court cases. Every time they ran a piece, they received plenty of feedback, he says, and it was all negative. "I started hearing 'What are you printing that crap for? Those people are just trying to take advantage. They're just gold-diggers. They resent Grace leaving, they're just looking for a free payday.'" It made some sense, he says. There was a lot of resentment directed at Grace when the corporation closed Libby's mine despite all the local efforts to keep things running. He felt obligated to mention these cases, but not to take it any further.

Then one day, Les Skramstad walked into Morris's office. "This town isn't safe," he proclaimed. He wasn't carrying any of the voluminous files, nothing of the vast document collection he and Gayla had amassed for their court cases. Morris thought he had a nut on his hands. "Well, that's not the right thing to say to me because right away you put me on the defensive." Morris paid Les no attention. Now he shakes his head. He knows his crew could have done more. Ultimately, however, he doesn't think it would have made any difference.

"There was no way to get this out in the open and get the EPA here. It never would have happened unless it happened the way it did. We probably would have been out of business if we'd done something like that."

It took an outsider, a big-shot, big-city journalist to crack through the silence that had engulfed Libby for so long. By the time Andrew Schneider turned up on Gayla Benefield's porch, she says, the asbestos people had just about gone hoarse trying to get someone's attention. "You talk about whistleblowers," she says, chuckling. "We had a whole damn marching band up here and it seemed like everyone was deaf. ... Maybe no one had the breath to blow loud enough."

Grace almost escaped the state without news of its deadly legacy in Libby going public. Then in 1999, the State decided it was time to pay back to Grace the remnants of the company's original $472,000 reclamation bond. All that was left by then was about $67,000. At this time, Gayla says, there was a great deal of disconnect between those in Libby who knew the horror Grace had perpetuated there and those who had no clue. The bond money was a drop in the bucket, but for the State to give it back when so many were dying was a final insult. She sent a letter of protest to the Department of Environmental Quality, which eventually found its way to the Helena office of the Montana Environmental Information Center (MEIC). This is where Schneider came in.

Schneider is a Pulitzer Prize–winning journalist, an itinerant reporter who had signed on as the special projects writer at the Seattle *Post Intelligencer*. In 1999 he traveled to Helena, Montana, to do a story about the reclamation of gold mines. Or that's what he told Gayla when he ended up in her kitchen. "He had come through checking on the old gold mines, and that's what he was doing here, just floating around the state." Schneider told Gayla he had walked into the office of the MEIC and asked the staff if anything interesting was going on. "They say, 'Well, yeah, Libby, W.R. Grace mine, deaths. ...' And Andy picked up on it."

When Schneider showed up at Gayla's front door with a photographer in tow, she was, she freely admits, intimidated. "He scared the pants off me. Gruff, actually," she says. First she took him to the mountain. "We turned up, started up Rainy Creek, and he was commenting on how beautiful the river was and all that, everything else. We pulled up to the tailings and he just sat there. 'How long has it been there?'

"'Ten years.'" Still worried about the jury pool, Gayla at first answered only the questions Schneider asked her directly. She thought she could keep Schneider to his reclamation story. But, she says, he knew what to look for.

At the junction of the mine road and the river, Schneider asked about the old loading facility. Gayla told him what it had been and added that some folks had turned it into a nursery.

"'Someone living there?'"

"'Yeah.'"

"Then coming across the bridge, he pointed to the ball field and says, 'What is that over there?' 'Well,' I says, 'that's the expanding plant, loading facility.' 'What's that?' 'Baseball fields.' 'When did they shut down?' I said, '1997.' He said, 'Oh my God.'"

Gayla invited Schneider to her house the next day to look at her files. He was astounded. He wanted to know if she had written her thesis on Grace, and where she had gone to college. "Nowhere," she told him.

"'Why do you have this?'"

Gayla replied, laughing, "'Hobby.' It was hard to gauge if he thought this was a story or not, or just a crazy woman." It was September 1999. Schneider made copies of her Grace library, then left town. Gayla didn't hear anything for a few months. Then one day in November he called.

"He called me just before [the story went to press] and said, 'Gayla, it's got two ways to go. I can take all my work and just trash it right now or release the story. If I release the story,' he says, 'things are going to change forever.'" Gayla gave it some thought. The state had been no help; the Helena EPA office useless as well. No other journalist had ever shown an interest: the local editor thought the asbestos victims were just a bunch of cranks. This story by Schneider might be their last best chance to save their community and might make it a safe place for her grandkids to grow up. "I said, 'No, the story's got to run.'"

By then, other writers had gotten wind of Schneider's project. The Kalispell *Daily Inter Lake*, which had refused to touch the issue for years, sent a writer to do a quickie weekend job and beat Schneider to publication by a day or two. A group of students from the university in Missoula were doing a classroom project on Libby as well. But it was Schneider's series, "An Uncivil Action," published the week before Thanksgiving 1999, that woke Libby from its long, dark nightmare.

For Libby, Schneider's series was a mirror, and what the towns-people saw when they looked at themselves through the lens of the outside world was not flattering. If they accepted the story as true, it meant evil had walked among them for decades and they had chosen to ignore it. It meant this company town had been betrayed by its company, and the possibility shook their worldview to its foundations. And it meant they, too, might die a very hard death. It was as if a mighty earthquake hit town on November 18, 1999, and split it into two along a fault line no one knew existed.

Libby Redux

Dillon, Montana, sits on the boundary of east and west. Sunk in the ground at the junction of two river valleys about 300 miles to the south of Libby, the small town is surrounded by both tree-covered hills and high plateaus. The vermiculite mine is about 13 miles out of town as the raven flies, and more like 23 miles by gravel road. In late July, balsamroot flowers line the first few miles of road out of town, blooming like feral sunflowers. Past the ceme-tery, a ranch and a farm or two, the road begins to glitter with ore from the local talc mine. The vermiculite mine itself is hidden to the west on a tree-covered hill, but from the top of a ridge one can visually follow the route all the way to town, along the road where the high school cross-country runners train, and along which the Utah-based Stansbury Holding Corporation hoped to haul out 50,000 tons of asbestos-contaminated vermiculite a year for twenty-five years.

Stansbury's plan to expand its relatively tiny 5-acre operation— small enough to be exempt from most state environmental laws— was all but approved by the Department of Environmental Quality (DEQ) in April 1999, seven months before the news about Libby came out. The plan would have gone through, too, if Seattle re-porter Andrew Schneider had not walked into the local Patagonia outlet store after his series on Libby was published.

"He comes up to me and says, 'So, doll, what do you think about having a vermiculite mine in your town?'" store manager Holly Miller recalls. "And I said, '*What?* What are you talking about?'"

In some ways Miller couldn't be more different than Benefield: proud to call herself an environmentalist, Miller gardens, raises llamas, and is a working artist. But like Gayla, Holly is a native Montanan, a grandmother, and a boundless fury rises in her voice when she considers the threat of asbestos poisoning to her children and grandchildren. "I have two granddaughters. I have a five-year-old and a three-year-old, and all the rest of it doesn't mean anything. You think about what those families in Libby are going through. It just boggles the mind to think this has been reviewed so carelessly."

"Carelessly" means that Montana's DEQ ran the mine expansion proposal through its least stringent review process, then gave the okay (pending receipt of a reclamation bond that never came) without addressing any of the issues that might have saved Libby its grief.

After Schneider clued her in, Miller did her homework. There was asbestos in Dillon's vermiculite—tremolite asbestos. And there were good reasons not to trust Stansbury. The company purchased the mine—with its expansion request pending before the state—in June 1999, and soon thereafter increased operations to 16 acres, in violation of the permit that limited it to 5 acres. Although the state required that the company post a $258,000 reclamation bond for its proposal to expand to 35 acres, DEQ official Warren McCullough says, Stansbury didn't send the money but began mining anyway.

Armed with this information, Miller got to work. She set out petitions at the Patagonia store and talked to everyone she knew about the mine. "I wrote a million letters. I wrote to the Denver EPA, the Washington EPA. I wrote every place I could think would have any kind of hope of assistance or at least consideration. Geez, you know, we don't know what we're even sitting on here."

Her persistence paid off: the DEQ agreed to reopen its decision to further public comment and held a hearing in Dillon one summer evening. "I called in all my cards," she says. "I said, 'Hey, I baby-sat for you when I was in seventh grade. I never asked you for any-thing, but I need you to be at that meeting. Come with whatever opinions you've got, but be at that meeting.'

"I'll tell you, the first hour of it, I had the most sinking feeling. The mayor wouldn't let anybody speak. First he let DEQ talk for the first half an hour, then the fat cat from Stansbury got up there. There wasn't any local representation." Stansbury brought in a Scottish expert, John Addison of the Institute for Occupational Medicine. Addison introduced himself by bragging that "the main reason I was invited here is my reputation for being extremely tough on asbestos." Addison picked up a fist-sized hunk of rock he claimed to have found up at the mine site that morning. He told the crowded room it was a crystalline-structured tremolite. "The dust from this would be no more harmful than the dust from any road stone quarry, any rock, any garden dust," he said. "No more harmful." He wasn't convinced Dillon had any fibrous tremolite at all. Though the DEQ had recently taken further ore samples from the site, and one of these had turned up with tremolite asbestos at 0.75 percent, Addison waved it off as sloppy fiber analysis. What some people call "asbestos," he said, are merely "chunky fibers which I consider not to be asbestos."

Addison talked for a good half hour before he yielded the floor. But when he did, the Benefields and Skramstads were there to clear out the hot air. They had driven down from Libby in the hopes of sparing their fellow Montanans some agony. "I've said that if this goes through," Gayla said, "we might as well be joined at the hip."

As they spoke, Miller says, the mood shifted. "Les stood up, and of course he had to sit on a table because of his breathing, he was so labored. I tell you, you could have heard a pin drop," Miller says. "All of a sudden, I think more than anything, these people put a face to statistics. Statistics are just numbers. But then when you see these people, it's a whole different movie. Gayla just said, 'I'm not here to tell any of you people what to do about this mine, but I am here to tell you that my folks are dead and we were told ex-actly the same things that these guys are saying right now.'"

It wasn't even one of her more articulate moments, but Gayla Benefield filled the room with the force of her presence. She urged the people of Dillon to make an informed decision and told them they could trust their safety to no one but themselves.

If it weren't for Libby grabbing national headlines, Miller says, no one would have noticed a little 35-acre vermiculite mine in Dillon—or cared. As it is, she still has a tough time convincing her neighbors that they don't need jobs that badly. "You'd think this would be the one time when people would stand up and say no," she says. "But it's not happening. People are really divided on the question. This is hurting our economy. That's always the thing that just drops me in my tracks. What does the economy have to do with this? I mean, we're talking about people dropping over dead."

NINE

Reckoning

"I'M SO SICK OF Gayla Benefield I could spit." The woman with a heavy Norwegian accent practically does spit out these words, and heads all around the room nodded in agreement. The governor is in town—Governor Judy Martz. She was elected as Marc Racicot's replacement when he left to work for the Republican National Committee. Martz spent the day touring Libby with Paul Peronard of the EPA, sat through three hours of testimony at a town meeting, and now can relax a bit with the people. Her people. The Chamber of Commerce organized a short meeting to debrief the governor at the end of the day, and they are pleading with her to put an end to the bad publicity their town has endured.

It is Martz's first public visit to Libby since winning the election nine months earlier, and the big issue on the table is whether or not Libby should become a Superfund site, a designation that would qualify the town for federal cleanup funds. The people at the chamber meeting are almost unilaterally opposed to the idea; they wince at every news report about Libby's asbestos problems and fear a Superfund designation will simply keep the story alive. Real estate agents are convinced that potential buyers won't be able to get loans for houses under the Superfund cloud, and cite anecdotal evidence that the local housing market has gone into a decline. Others fear the government will come onto their property whether they like it or not, declare their homes and businesses un-livable, and maybe even send them the cleanup bill.

But the governor's support for Superfund is crucial, Peronard tells me the next morning. The EPA emergency response team has been operating in Libby for more than eighteen months and has spent $6 million; the provision under which they worked was meant for much shorter-term projects: 12 months, $2 million at the most. While his immediate superiors are supportive, someone in Washington, D.C., could easily find reason to pull the plug on the operation. Superfund is the perfect place for Libby. Congress enacted the law in 1980 to provide a mechanism to deal with the nation's worst toxic waste sites, places that would likely never get cleaned up but for federal intervention. Lawmakers funded the program over the years to the tune of $15.2 billion, though since the authorizing legislation lapsed in 1994, and President George W. Bush has indicated his intention simply to let the fund bleed to death financially, its long-term viability is rather doubtful. But Peronard, ever the optimist, is nevertheless pushing for Libby's listing.

The EPA has only once in its history declared a Superfund site over a governor's objection, and Peronard tells me that it is not going to happen here. Governor Martz has to give her approval. If she doesn't, the EPA has three choices: continue to operate as an emergency team, ask for money from Congress, or walk away. "It would be a shame. We shouldn't walk away from this," he says. But it could happen, and if the EPA leaves, no one else is standing in line to help.

By the time of Martz's visit, the battle lines are clearly drawn. On one side are members of Libby's business community and Grace; on the other, the EPA and Grace's victims. They skirmish over every issue: meeting formats, analytical techniques, standards for the cleanup, even access to the mine site. The final major battle, however, is Superfund. With it, Libby has a future. Without it, no one knows.

In the months after the EPA team arrived, Gayla became their not-so-silent partner, playing the political and public relations whiz to Peronard's and Weis's science guy routine. But the relationship came neither quickly nor easily. It was, she says, an issue of trust.

"I have learned when it comes to this situation not to trust. At some point I had to make up my mind and I had to trust some agency. But it took awhile. They had to earn their trust. I think they had to come out publicly and say, 'We dropped the ball. We made a mistake. God, what can we do to help?' They had to keep coming back to me before I accepted them. I didn't accept them as my saviors."

Peronard made that apology, then asked Gayla if he could bring the entire EPA team out to her house. "And it was like, 'Why?'

"And Paul said, 'Well, you know, if this would go Superfund, the state, the company that did the dirty work, would do it and the state will …'

"'Well,' I said, 'just forget it. My gut feeling is the company knew what they were doing and the state let it happen.'

"Paul said, 'How can you say that?'"

That's when Gayla brought her files out. "I had a starter kit of the evidence. It was sort of my own combination of things I'd picked up. And I sent those back to Denver with them. That was his first indoctrination into the bowels of Grace.

"Paul said he has never been so depressed in his life. He came out here that first week thinking he was going to meet a real crazy lady with the wild hair," she says, laughing. "Once he did just an initial overview and looked at the documents, and saw the sickness and talked to the people, he said he left here and was so depressed. 'Oh my God, what's happened to that community?' I mean, what did we consider normal all those years? Well, it was just the miners. Like they're expendable, they worked there, they deserved to die."

From then on, Gayla was an honorary member of the crew, providing the benefit of nearly sixty years' experience of living under the shadow of Grace's mountain. Peronard, she says, still thought he could work something out with the company. "He said, 'We've dealt with some terrible companies. I'm sure we can deal with them. We've been on some really bad Superfund sites.'"

Gayla knew better, but decided she could work with this earnest young man anyway. She began by prodding the scientists to use more modern analytical techniques. When Peronard sent the first round of samples to Denver for analysis, Gayla called him up.

"'Paul, what methods are you using?'

"'Well, phase contrast microscopy.'

"I said, 'Paul, W.R. Grace was using that same method in 1973. Don't you have a bigger microscope down there?'

"'Well, yeah.'

"I said, 'Don't you have a *really big* microscope down there? Give us the benefit of top of the line of what you've got.'"

One of the samples that had come out clean under phase contrast microscopy told the whole story when put under the transmission electron microscope: "Paul put it under the big microscope and it blew him away," she says. "Suddenly, it's a bundle of hundreds of fibers. All it took was that one picture."

Gayla became the EPA's entree into the suspicious community. Townspeople started taking them up on the offer to just drop by the office and talk things over. The maps went up on the walls; the sampling crews began to target their spots more efficiently. The cleanup was on.

As Peronard and Weis focused on the technical aspects, Gayla worked the phones and the media. When Montana's sole congressional representative, Republican Denny Rehberg, organized for a roundtable discussion of whether Libby should become a Superfund site—but neglected to include on the panel anyone who supported the idea—she made the phone calls and badgered the congressman's people until they apologized and fixed things. A natural-born speaker, Gayla rivaled Peronard for her skill with the press, appearing on the Discovery Channel, *Dateline*, and 20/20, talking to journalists from the *New York Times*, *People Magazine*, and *All Things Considered*. Her granddaughter Amy's graduation even made television when CBS insisted on filming that day. "I had to get up at 6 A.M.! This is the sound stage; 6 A.M. they had to come in and set up. And I said, 'Don't even wake me up.' By then I knew the crews. I just said, 'Holler when you guys get ready to shoot.'"

Paul Peronard may have been in charge, but he wouldn't have gotten there without Gayla. She was the conductor of the whole grand scheme. So I pay attention when she tells me one morning, "You go down to La Casa de Amigos. Stop in there in the morning and you're going to hear anything you want to hear. Some of them just speak out. They say that this is completely staged, it's not happening, we're just trying to destroy the community. You really should go down there. I need to have ears down there."

Libby is an unlikely place for a Mexican restaurant, about as far
north of Mexico as one can get in the American West. But La Casa
de Amigos restaurant on California Avenue is a modern landmark.
At 10 A.M. every weekday, an exclusive group of businessmen and
bureaucrats gather for their morning coffee. About a dozen of
them show up on each of the two days I stop by: all white men,
ranging from middle age on up. They include an auto mechanic, a
college president, a real estate agent, a lawyer, and a state senator.
On some days, Grace spokesperson Alan Stringer appears. He
doesn't stand out; he is just another one of the guys. It's a friendly
crowd, and they make a stranger feel welcome. "If you're a reporter, we'll talk to you," one says. I take a seat at the end of the
table, pour a little milk into the cup of coffee they have given me,
and start listening.

They rib each other mostly. This group—or their fathers and
grandfathers—began meeting in 1941 at the now-defunct Rexall
Drug Store. They admit Libby has a problem, but feel Gayla is self-
aggrandizing, that things will take care of themselves, that their
community has been portrayed one-sidedly as a poisoned town.
They ask for my take on the situation, and it's not fair to equivo-
cate as I want to know what lies in their hearts as well. I tell them
how I walked around town the previous night breathing the fra-
grant air, enjoying the pretty yards filled with lilies, yellow
columbine, hardy old rosebushes, and tried to reconcile the beauty
and serenity with the horror that has happened here. They seem
satisfied that I find the situation complex, and as the gathering
breaks up, one man offers to take me to neighboring Troy later that
week with his family for the Fourth of July celebration.

Individually, local businesspeople are reluctant to talk on the
record. The few who have spoken with the press usually feel
burned by the results. So it takes some convincing for Jack
DeShazer Jr. to agree to an interview, but he finally gives in. Jack
is in an awkward position. As co-owner of a successful real estate
agency—billboards announce his business on all the major roads
into town—DeShazer believes the publicity surrounding Libby's
asbestos problems is a drag on the economy, and could end up

costing him personally. But his father, the man for whom he is named, worked at the mine and brought his family to live in the company cabins on Rainy Creek Road. His mother and father have been diagnosed, his sister too. An athletic man, Jack runs 5 miles three days a week and refuses to be tested. But he is friends with Gayla's daughter, Jenan Swenson, who cleans house for his parents. He coaches her daughter's basketball team and gets an earful whenever Jen feels the need to proselytize the gospel according to Gayla. So while he, like the rest of the Chamber of Commerce crowd, bemoans the bad press Libby has been getting, he catches himself disparaging the asbestos victims.

"The media and people that are trying to get something out of their disability—there's a lot of people making it sound worse than it is," he says. "But if you're sick or your parents are sick or something like that, obviously you're angry."

DeShazer says the real estate market isn't large enough so that anyone can draw any sort of statistically meaningful conclusions, but it's hard to doubt that his gut instinct—that the market has been hit hard—is right on. "The biggest effect is lack of people wanting to move here," he says. "I mean, it doesn't matter to most people if they live in Kalispell or Eureka or Thompson Falls or Troy or Libby. And if you've read something bad about the air here, why would you even consider it? So you know, like hits on the Internet? That kind of thing has been drastically reduced. And less activity means lesser prices." He has the anecdotes: houses that went for far less than they would have before the news broke, houses that normally would have sold but are simply sitting there, other deals that fell apart all together. While riverside and lakefront properties are still selling well, and he has no trouble finding buyers for exclusive land bordered by the national forest, DeShazer says even those people "expect to pay less money if they buy it here versus if they buy it in Whitefish or Kalispell." For proof he sends me to appraiser Verle Howell.

Howell has hard numbers. "A more accurate way of looking at the situation is the marketing time," he says. "Last year it was 210 days, this year over 300 days on average, that it takes to sell a house." Volume is down as well. In recent years, he says, Libby averaged around 120 houses sold. As of the end of October 2001, only 79 homes had sold. And as the EPA considers putting Libby on the national Superfund list, the realtors fear that what's left of the market will plummet.

As an appraiser, part of Howell's job is to determine whether Libby's market is increasing or declining. A declining market, he says, is the kiss of death. "When that happens, the secondary loan markets won't touch Libby loans, and banks won't be able to make the loans, and people won't be able to buy or sell." Also, Howell says, he's afraid local realtors will have to count on the EPA to go house to house and declare each building safe before a sale can be finalized. "They're going to have to change the rules a little bit."

The problem with that, DeShazer says, is that none of his colleagues trust Peronard. "One thing is, my gosh, look at all the people who are talking to him. He's an important guy, you know. Everybody has an ego. It's part of what is going on," he says. "But he does have good qualities, and that's what makes him dangerous. You can't dislike him. The charisma he has. The media like that and it cost us, it really did."

Furthermore, DeShazer says, things like federal toxics laws are unfamiliar territory for the average Libby businessperson, and so they are having a hard time communicating with Peronard. "I asked him four times, 'What are you going to do as far as cleaning up the tremolite out of residential houses?' And he went on for ten minutes each time ... and never said a damn thing. All of those people—they will not answer a pointed question, yes or no. It's intimidating and you have to sound ignorant not to understand. He's talking in terms you don't understand."

"He actually cares," DeShazer admits. "He just doesn't care enough in the right direction."

It's not a stretch to say the business community has been victimized here as well, dealt an economic blow not measurable by X-ray machines and not compensable by jury verdicts. But in the wake of the publicity, the vocal businesspeople have been more inclined to blame the messenger for Libby's mess than the real culprit.

It is as if the entire town is progressing collectively through the stages of grief, hospice worker Laura Sedler tells me. Until recently a lot of people were stuck in denial. "They said it wasn't really true, it hadn't really happened. That the people who were asbestos victims, the 'Asbestos People' as they were called, were after the money; that that was the only thing that was going on. They were trying to sue Grace to get rich. Just all these various forms of denial. It's fascinating, from the point of view of a sociologist, to watch."

Sedler is the inheritor of Dr. Richard Irons's pilot project. Though she has dedicated her life to taking care of the people here, Sedler is not one of them. She grew up in San Diego and moved here after her sister married a Libby boy. As such, she is intimate with Libby's sickness but also removed from it. She lives, literally, in a different world: to get to the home she shares with her husband, one must drive almost to the Idaho state line, take a right up the Yaak River, and turn off on a side road that, if followed all the way, eventually returns to Libby. The yard of their A-frame is wild with flowers and birds. We sip tea and listen to the creek rushing by. "In some ways it's really good," she says. "I'm sure it's really good for me because I don't have to eat, sleep, and breathe it. That's kind of literal there."

In her hospice work, Sedler has found the social repercussions to be as forceful as the physical illness. Her clients have had to deal not only with the mechanics of their disease but with being ostracized as well. "The biggest issue was their feelings of betrayal by their community, that they were being blamed, that they were victims and they were being blamed for what's happening. They were very angry; they were very hurt." In response, she and her colleagues started a support group for asbestos victims, a place where people could work through all the implications of their disease. "We had a guy who came to the support group. He came from [out of town] because he had nobody to talk to over there. He was afraid he was going to lose his job if they found out he'd been diagnosed. He was completely undercover as far as having asbestosis. He didn't even tell people he had grown up in Libby. He drove all the way over for the support group. And he was a diesel truck driver, he was a teamster. And at the first meeting he kept saying, 'No, I'm not angry. Things happen, blah blah blah.' And toward the end of the meeting he goes, 'But if it ever meant that I couldn't work, I don't what I'd do. I'd be angry. I wouldn't even want to go on living if I couldn't work.'

"And some of the other people in the group were pointing out that you're driving a truck and you're exposed to that diesel all the time. But that's a hard choice for somebody who's grown up in a small town, and he's been a Teamster since he was nineteen, twenty years old. He loves his work—one of those people who their work is their life. And you know, we're kind of saying, 'Well, maybe you should go to school and learn to do stuff on a computer.' How do people make those changes? Some people do it.

"We get a lot of bargaining," she says. "Like that guy saying, 'Well, it's okay as long as it doesn't affect my job.' That's bargaining. Or when sometimes people do it with God. They'll say, 'You know, God, just let me live until my granddaughter's wedding, and then I'm okay with this.' Or the one we heard a lot in group was 'If W.R. Grace would just apologize, then it would be okay.'"

By all indications, Grace is not going to apologize to anyone.

As the news reports filtered out into the wider world—including Andrew Schneider's counting of 200 death certificates from patients he believed had been killed by Grace's "nuisance dust"—company executives expressed great concern and pledged their cooperation. The company's first public statement bore the headline "Grace urges state of Montana and U.S. EPA to move quickly to address reported health concerns in Libby, Montana." The press release quoted Grace vice president William Corcoran, who said his heart was with Libby. "Our concern is that the people of Libby have many questions and few answers. … W.R. Grace is committed to complete cooperation with your efforts and offers to help you in any way we can."

About a week later, Grace CEO Paul Norris added his two cents: "Agency oversight reports on the mine reclamation project were positive. We are interested in learning the facts as quickly as possible so that we know what steps, if any, need to be taken." Within a month, Grace pledged to donate $250,000 a year to the local St. John's Lutheran Hospital, to set up a medical plan to care for those who had been made sick by the mine, and to pay for asbestos health screenings. The first two promises were greeted with wary acceptance. The federal Agency for Toxic Substances and Disease Registry, however, decided to pick up the tab for the screenings. What they found astounded nearly everyone: 30 percent of the 6,144 adults who volunteered for the first round of testing had lung abnormalities, and 18 percent of those were judged to have "probable" asbestos-related disease. Though there may be statistical adjustments to make because only half the community was tested, the results mean that at least every fifth person in this county of 12,000 is walking around with death in his or her lungs.

Furthermore, 5 percent of those with lung abnormalities had no known exposure pathway to Grace's tremolite: they never worked at the mine and didn't live with anyone who had. They never played in the vermiculite piles; they never played Little League. They had no Zonolite insulation in their homes, and they never attended a kegger at the turnout on Rainy Creek Road. They simply lived in Libby.

The medical plan, too, is full of loopholes. One snag is the plan's longevity: while Libby can expect to see new cases of asbestos-related diseases for the next forty years, Grace retained discretion to cancel the plan at its whim. Grace's asbestos victims say they don't expect that fund will exist much past the end of the corporation's bankruptcy proceedings, if that long. A second problem is that Grace gets to decide who qualifies and who doesn't. Everything went smoothly at first, then midway through 2002, Dr. Black and his staff noticed that nearly two-thirds of those who had recently applied for medical coverage—seventeen out of twenty-seven—were turned down. Grace spokesperson Alan Stringer would say only that the rejected applicants didn't show sufficient evidence of having an asbestos-related disease.

The EPA responded to Grace's overtures by entering negotiations over the town's cleanup. "In retrospect," Peronard told reporters, "it turned out to be a rather nonproductive negotiation process and that's really the rub." The agency had test results by early spring 2000 showing that the Raintree Nursery and expansion plant next to the baseball fields were dangerously contaminated. Grace balked, however, and said that if the agency wanted Grace to help clean these spots, they'd have to order it to do so. "We don't want to give up our rights," Alan Stringer told the *Western News*. So Peronard's team issued the order for Grace to clean the expansion plant property next to the baseball fields. The EPA decided to take care of the nursery itself and bill Grace for the job.

This task was probably Grace's last best chance for goodwill with the community. The EPA specified that Grace was to clean out all the old buildings on the 6-acre site and excavate 18 inches of topsoil. The company hired contractors and the work was done—or so they said. Les Skramstad decided to do his own inspection of the job and came back with a mason jar full of vermiculite he had scraped off the ground with Norita's gardening trowel. Grace spokesperson Alan Stringer was incensed. "It is entirely possible that [Les] collected that vermiculite from the export plant, but it wasn't there when Grace completed the clean up. That is simply not possible," Stringer wrote in a guest editorial for the *Western News*, all but accusing Les of planting the ore there.

Les was, to put it mildly, beside himself at being called a liar in the newspaper. He rang up editor Roger Morris to set the record straight. Morris says, "Called me at home early in the morning. He says, 'Roger, I didn't make this up. I didn't spike the place with vermiculite. Will you meet with me?' And I said, 'Sure, Les.' And I got here in the morning and he was sitting here waiting for me. He wasn't supposed to be here until an hour later. I says, 'Boy, you're jumping to go, ain't ya?' And he says, 'Yep.' He says, 'Come on, we'll get in my truck and I'll drive you.'

"We went up to the edge of one of the buildings and he says, 'This is what I'm talking about.' He climbed down in there and started scraping loose vermiculite. And then he pulls a board off and it's just caked in there with spiderwebs over it and cobwebs. So nobody had touched it. And he filled baggie after baggie up with it. And then he took me inside the building and the wood inside the building was just embedded with it. You could see it sparkling in there.

"And he had told me about this ahead of time. I think it was a big mistake, public-relation-wise, at least to me it is. I worked four years in public relations: they left the rope hanging inside the building that the kids used to swing off the balcony into the vermiculite piles. The rope was still hanging there."

THINGS WERE ABOUT TO GET WORSE. After the mine closed in 1990, the property was sold to a group called the Kootenai Development Company, the partners of which included Jack Wolter, Grace's man in charge of reclamation after the mine closed. After the EPA came to town, Grace bought out a two-thirds majority of KDC on the quiet, regaining ownership of the mine site as well as land next to and across the river from the Parkers' nursery. Grace announced this to the EPA on July 18, 2000, and proclaimed that the agency was banned from both properties. At about this time, Peronard declared Grace to be "the most difficult company I've ever worked with." The EPA had to apply for a warrant to get on the land, and after the company responded by granting very limited access, the agency filed a lawsuit against Grace. The judge, Donald Molloy of the U.S. District Court in Missoula, was not amused.

In court, Grace argued that the EPA ought to pay for the privilege of entering its land to sample and test the dust and air, and to bury old mine waste up on the mountain, as was the agency's plan. Grace objected to the latter in particular, saying it would give the EPA precedent to dump toxic waste wherever it chose. Molloy was about as riled as a federal judge can get. "Defendants foresee dire consequences for the playgrounds of tender young schoolchildren, defenseless against the vicissitudes of EPA discretion. ... Grace should have acknowledged this concern for the public long ago in the sordid history of asbestos and its harmful effects. ...

"The conclusion is as plain to see as the East Front of the Rocky Mountains," Molloy wrote in dismissing another of Grace's arguments. More than sixteen months after Grace pledged its "complete cooperation" with the EPA, the agency was finally allowed back on the mine site under court order. But Grace hadn't used up all its weapons yet. Less than two weeks later, the great multinational corporation declared itself broke.

The move left Libby's victims—now shut out of court—wondering how a company with sales exceeding $5.5 billion each year through the first half of the 1990s could count only $1.5 billion in annual revenue by 1997. According to company officials, Grace's financial problems were all about asbestos: a broken court system, a sudden influx of asbestos cases—many of them "unmeritorious" claims brought by perfectly healthy people. Furthermore, Grace was carrying an increasingly heavy load of the nation's asbestos lawsuits as other companies went under. Johns-Manville led the pack in 1982, to be followed by twenty-six more companies by the turn of the century, according to the "W.R. Grace Bankruptcy Newsletter," published by the Bankruptcy's Creditor's Service. As each company failed, asbestos victims across the nation (mostly construction workers exposed to asbestos products from a wide array of sources) had fewer and fewer places to go for compensation. *Fortune* magazine reported that the lawsuits numbered 570,000 as of March 2002. It was the resulting domino effect, which caused a reported 81 percent increase in lawsuits filed against Grace in 2000, that pushed Grace under. "We believe that the state court system for dealing with asbestos claims is broken, and that Grace cannot effectively defend itself against unmeritorious claims," Grace CEO Paul Norris was quoted as saying in the bankruptcy newsletter. "Until recently, Grace was able to settle claims through direct negotiations. The filings of claims had stabilized and annual cash flows were manageable and fairly predictable."

In fact, however, Grace officers appear to have been preparing for Chapter 11 long before their caseload increased so dramatically. The drastic decrease in Grace's sales numbers *was* about asbestos, but it appears to have had little to do with healthy people scamming the court system. In a series of complicated transactions, Grace began in the mid-1990s to secrete away its profits for the purpose of protecting them from asbestos plaintiffs. "Grace had depleted its multibillion-dollar status in the late 1990s by two actions," Kalispell attorney Allan McGarvey explains. "First, it made distributions to its shareholders. ... Once the shareholders have the money, the corporation has lost the money and it is no longer available to satisfy the liabilities of the corporation.

"Second is a transaction called a spin-off. Corporation A can create a subsidiary (B) to hold part of its assets. Corp A holds all the shares of the Subsidiary B. Next the Corp A simply gives its shares in the subsidiary to its own shareholders, with the result that the shareholders now own two companies (A and B). As a result, A no longer owns B or any of B's assets."

Grace used this tactic twice, first spinning off in 1996 the National Medical Care company (now known as Fresenius Medical Care Holdings), and a year later a packaging company called Cryovac. In that case, Corporation A was the original W.R. Grace and Corporation B was Cryovac. Cryovac was a wholly owned Grace subsidiary, a company that invented shrink-wrap. In 1997, Grace announced it was selling Cryovac to a separate company called Sealed Air, which makes bubble wrap. It was a sweet deal for shareholders, turning Sealed Air from a company turning $800 million in annual revenue to one pulling in $2.5 billion, the *New York Times* reported. In return Grace received $1.2 billion in cash from Cryovac, which Grace planned to use "to pay down substantially all its debt," according to a company press release. And the whole thing was tax-free, the *Times* reported, because Grace shareholders would own a majority—63 percent—of Sealed Air. Grace said its liabilities would remain with the remnant Grace corporation, now worth only $1.5 billion in annual sales. "This was a great chance to split the packaging company away from the asbestos liabilities holding down our stock multiple," Grace chairman Albert J. Costello told the *Times* reporter.

Grace's filing was particularly cruel for Libby, attorney Roger Sullivan explains. While the nation's tradesmen have the option of seeking recompense from any of the remaining companies whose asbestos products they were exposed to, Libby victims can turn only to Grace. And Grace has bigger creditors to worry about than the petty tort claims of fisherman Royce Ryan and his former neighbors. Topping its list of creditors, for instance, is Chase Manhattan Bank, to whom Grace owes more than a half billion dollars.

The Kalispell lawyers are part of several class action suits arising from Grace's actions in Libby: one would protect those who have not yet been diagnosed with asbestos-related disease when they become sick in the future, a second would hold Grace responsible for the cost of the environmental cleanup in and around Lincoln County, and a third seeks money for removal of Zonolite attic insulation nationwide. But in terms of individual asbestos lawsuits, Libby ranks low. After informing me that no one from Grace would consent to an interview on the topic, spokesperson Greg Euston says that Grace had, as of November 2001, 150,000 asbestos lawsuits outstanding, of which only 180 were related to Libby. "That's 0.07 percent," he says.

Although Grace's creditors are trying to "pierce the corporate veil" (legal parlance for getting to the money Grace protected with those spin-offs) and have filed suit to reverse both transactions, Libby's lawyers are not optimistic. First, McGarvey says, lawyers have to prove the spin-offs were fraudulent, and they can only do so on narrow grounds. "Generally there must be some kind of showing of insolvency at the time of the distribution or spin-off," he says. "Second, there must be a target to recover the transferred assets. In this case, both the distributions and the spin-offs were transfers to the shareholders. Obviously, it is very difficult to attempt to reverse a transfer to hundreds of thousands of shareholders."

With such powerful creditors standing in line in front of Libby's plaintiffs, Sullivan says, his clients are likely to get the leftover scraps. "Here W.R. Grace caused these individuals to endure these most unimaginable diseases and deaths. If W.R. Grace walks away from that debt paying pennies on the dollar, who's going to pay? You are. The American public is. The American taxpayer will. And in my estimation that's outrageous if there are assets that should be properly available to fund those liabilities."

But even as Grace's bankruptcy filing made it painfully clear that the corporation could not be counted on to pay for Libby's cleanup, there were townspeople who clung to the hope that the company they'd trusted for so long would not betray them.

GOVERNOR MARTZ ARRIVES early enough in the morning to beat the summer heat that has been plaguing Libby in 2001. She flies into the tiny airport south of town and is escorted by a caravan of press and police to her first stop at the old expansion plant next to the ball fields. Paul Peronard tells Martz that the company's cleanup was inadequate, to put it mildly: passersby could still see the telltale sparkle of vermiculite lying in a ditch and falling out from under the building foundations. Martz listens to Peronard's spiel, then everyone begins to move on to the next stop, when a petite, middle-aged blonde woman grabs the governor's attention. Judy Burnett and her husband, Mel, are the current tenants of the old expansion plant; they run a retail lumber business here. Judy tries to tell the governor how difficult Grace has been to work with. "Our kids and grandkids have been exposed since '89. We had a huge business down here we had to move. ..."

"What's the bottom line? What are you saying?" the governor interrupts.

"I'm saying Grace is rotten," she says. Mel steps in. "They've fought us every minute to save themselves money."

Martz, a lanky but powerfully built woman known more for her physical strength than her intellectual prowess (she once competed as an Olympic speed skater), clearly feels ambushed and is not sure what to say to these people. "Where's Paul? I thought the EPA would direct you to relocate."

"The EPA directed Grace to relocate us, and Grace fought us every step of the way," Judy Burnett says. "They wanted to push us out in the streets. If we really let them do the cleanup, we can't let them treat homeowners around town like they've treated us. If it weren't for the EPA, we'd be out in the street." Burnett points to some sealed dumpsters across the dirt lot where, she says, Grace was to have placed their equipment after cleaning it. "Our equipment and tools are just thrown in there, and you open the boxes and everything is still covered in dust."

Next on the agenda is a visit to the high school track on the other side of town. Moon-suited workers have dug up the running track, which encircles the football field; it was paved with asbestos-laden mine tailings through most of the 1970s. Peronard tells the governor that the EPA divided the school grounds into a grid and sampled to 3 feet deep from every third grid. On a map he points to the yellow and red dots in a discrete oval that indicate asbestos where Grace laid down mine tailings for the track. Off to the side, the tennis courts carry traces as well. The company apparently used the courts as a staging ground, a place to pile up the contaminated tailings before laying the track. Peronard tells the governor they're finding asbestos readings at 5 to 30 percent, but that it seems to be confined to the track and the tennis courts. The agency is in the process of removing about 9,000 cubic yards of contaminated debris and soil. The roar of machinery is constant; a parade of dump trucks hauls contaminated debris from the school grounds through downtown Libby, up Rainy Creek Road (now closed to the public because of all the dust this traffic is raising) to the mine site where the waste is being buried.

Governor Martz is under the impression that if the asbestos, wherever it's found, is simply left alone, no one is in any danger. Peronard responds by quoting his colleague, toxicologist Chris Weis: "The activity drives the exposure," he says. If you dig a swimming pool, if you tear down the wrong dirt road on a four-wheeler raising dust, if you put a ceiling fan in your bathroom or install a sprinkler system for your lawn, you could be asking for trouble.

The start of football season is only a few weeks off, and the business community is starting to get nervous that opening day kickoff will need to be postponed. "They haven't mowed the lawn out there since last June, the last day of school it happened," one man complains to his fellow Chamber of Commerce members at the end of the day. "Football season starts here in three or four weeks and we've got a football field that looks like a dump zone. If they say there's no economic loss, what about the loss to my business on Friday and Saturday night, people stopping in and eating dinner before and after? And I'm sympathetic in a way. I mean, I'm a double victim. I worked up there; I have it. I hopefully will never die from it. And maybe a lot more people may never die from it.

"Ten percent of us in Lincoln County probably have asbestos. That's a thousand, 1,200 people. But should we take down the other 9,000 people with us? Because we don't want to look at our community and grow in a positive direction? We don't need to jump into something here that's going to take down our economic community."

The governor's last stop this morning is the old loading facility and former home of Lerah and Mel Parker's Raintree Nursery at the junction of the river and Rainy Creek Road. The property is enclosed in a series of fences delineating a succession of neutral zones where workers suit up before getting into the bad stuff. Today the place is crawling with heavy machinery, guys in hard hats, men in moonsuits. After Grace's pathetic job on the ball fields, the EPA took over the cleanup. Peronard explains what his agency is doing here: digging 12 feet deep in some places and hauling all the contaminated waste to the mine site to be buried.

The governor asks if she can go up to see the mine, but Peronard turns her down. With all the dump truck traffic raising dust on the road, he says, it's just too dangerous. She doesn't seem to understand, so he explains. "The stuff is not that easily controlled," he says. "You could smash a piece of vermiculite and you don't get shards. It just sorta disappears in a cloud of dust." He stops and looks up at the reporters scribbling notes. "Umm ... you should do this wearing a respirator," he adds quickly.

When Peronard finishes, it's Lerah Parker's turn to talk to the governor, scrapbook in hand. A minute into her presentation, she breaks down sobbing. The governor attempts to comfort her, putting an arm out, but Lerah pulls away and Peronard takes over again. Off to the side she tearfully answers reporters' questions until her husband shows up, when she breaks down again. "I just lost it," she tells Mel, accepting his embrace.

After lunch, the governor is scheduled to attend a town meeting. Gayla Benefield spent most of the last week orchestrating this event, making sure the speakers cover every essential point. For three hours, members of the packed audience at the American Legion hall stand at the microphone and use their three minutes to tell the governor about their families and their heartaches. More than one person chide the governor for taking so long to make this trip, seven months after she took office. Helen Bundrock is upset about a comment Martz made to a reporter that the atmosphere in Libby was too emotional. "Emotion is all I have left," she says. "It's not emotions that are dangerous, but lack of them." Gayla's daughter, Jenan Swenson, reads a poem she wrote. The school superintendent tells the governor the district has had to cut a half million dollars from its budget this year, and expects to do the same in 2002 because of a loss of enrollment. Even Norita Skramstad, who normally shuns the limelight, takes a few moments to ask the governor to consider the fate of people like her grown children. "Younger people are being diagnosed, and what are they going to do when they can't work? Grace's medical plan is only there so long as they're solvent." Nearly everyone urges the governor not to trust Grace with the cleanup of their town, to give the go-ahead for a Superfund designation.

It is an exhausting three hours, and at the end Martz takes the floor for a few moments. She has pledged neutrality on the Superfund subject and has claimed to have an open mind. But the words that come out of her mouth shock the assemblage to silence. "Quit criticizing, quit condemning, quit complaining," she says, as if scolding a whiny child. "You ask where your government's been? We're here. Laying blame will get us nowhere. You'll still be sick, you'll still be losing business."

By the time Martz arrives at the small Chamber of Commerce gathering in a conference room at the Venture Inn motel next to the cemetery, everyone is tired. The governor has only a few minutes to spend here before jetting off to Helena, and she uses the time to reassure the business community that while they may feel alienated in their own town, she has their interests at heart. "If they run the businesses out of town, where do they buy groceries? Where do they get their car fixed? Do they want to run to Kalispell to do all that? Because that's what happens when you start ostracizing people," she says. Martz encourages those gathered to write to her as a group so they will remain anonymous individually.

In the months after Martz was elected, little she said could have reassured Libby's victims. When characterizing her administration's strategy for Montana's economic revival, she announced that she planned to be the "lapdog of industry." She taunted at every turn those of her constituents who considered themselves environmentalists. So when she announced four months after her Libby visit that she had made a decision on Superfund, Grace's victims braced themselves for the worst.

What happened next surprised nearly everyone: Martz said that not only would she support naming Libby to the Superfund's National Priorities List, she would use her one "silver bullet" to ask the EPA to expedite the process as well. Almost no one was expecting it—not even Gayla. "It's rather unbelievable isn't it?" she e-mailed me. "I almost got up at sunrise today to check and see if the sun rose in the west!"

Gayla speculates that some of the governor's fellow Republicans influenced her decision. Democratic state attorney general Mike McGrath as well urged the governor to go Superfund; as of August 2001, nearly 200 people left adrift by Grace's bankruptcy had filed notice of their intent to sue the state instead. McGrath pointed out that in its shaky financial state, Montana can't bear the burden of these lawsuits, or of the entire cleanup, by itself. And with Grace in bankruptcy court, he said, the company is unlikely to be of much help.

But in fact there were two people who were not surprised at the governor's apparent change of heart: Les Skramstad and Paul Peronard. This is because while Gayla was quoted in a local newspaper as saying "Fuck you" to Martz, Skramstad started talking to Martz. "I guess I wasn't surprised because I had talked to her about it several different times," Les says. "She just kept telling me, 'I'm going to study that.' She didn't say yes or no. She just said she was going to check into it. And I think after she did, she determined that we really did have a serious problem here.

"Now a lot of people are saying it was a political thing, that they'd taken a poll or something in the state and everybody figured that we should have it. Well, heck, that was the feeling I think for quite a while before she'd done it. But I talk to her now on a fairly regular basis. She calls me and I call her and we visit for a while."

For her part the governor says she simply meant what she said: she had an open mind all along. "My experience has been that the private sector does things better," she says. "I looked into things, read a lot, talked to people, and realized this situation was different." Peronard's promise to have Libby cleaned up within three years of a Superfund designation and her contact with Les Skramstad made the difference. "Les reminds me of my father, actually," she says. "He wasn't confrontational. He's a good honest man. ... So I listened to him, looked into what he told me, and found out what he was telling me was right." His story, she says, broke her heart: "I don't know how you can listen to those stories from the people up there and not have your heart broken."

Peronard thinks the governor simply used her common sense. "My boss is always fond of saying, 'If you show people the logical and reasonable decisions, they're hard put to make a bad one.' And I just think it was a matter of she just spent enough time looking at it, hearing from enough folks, that she couldn't help but sort of come to that feeling that hey, look, this is the only way for us to move forward."

JENAN SWENSON STOPS HER CAR at the top of the DeShazers' driveway. The dogs haven't seen her yet, so she sits watching the reflection of the elderly couple's decorative windmill flash in the downstairs window. No one is in the yard; trees shade the abandoned garden, Jack Sr.'s pride for so many years. It's relatively good dirt, right next to the Kootenai River. But through the years the trees grew too high and blocked out the sun. By the time they'd had the trees cut, Jack was too sick to replant the garden. And now they realize the whole yard is likely contaminated—the soil that grew the food that fed their family is probably full of asbestos, and like everyone else in town they are advised not to stir things up.

Jack's plastic chair sits empty in its usual place next to his old blue Chevy pickup, about 50 feet from the door. If he had to leave the house, he could get this far before needing to rest. Margaret, his wife, uses an oxygen tank about two-thirds of the time. She has tried to give up smoking but can't. All they have energy for these days are small gestures for each other, sitting together, laughing at the Lone Ranger on television. This is why Jenan is here—to clean up the house for them. She rests her forehead on the steering wheel for a moment, pushing from her mind the kids and work, the pounding memories compounded by the unusual summer heat. Exhaling slowly, she puts the car in reverse, checking the road for people coming fast around the bend, and backs out. She just can't do it today. She will call Margaret later and apologize.

Margaret. Her grandmother's name. It is nearly six years since she died, since Jenan; her mother, Gayla; her aunt Eva; and her sisters organized their every waking minute for seventeen months around the schedule of a dying woman. Not until she saw her grandma in a casket did Jenan realize how much of Margaret was stolen by the disease. The energetic, independent woman she had known as a second mother turned into a demanding old witch who could control nothing in her life but her ability to order her care-takers around. The sight of Margaret in the coffin was a shock. With the lines of pain, distress, and the struggle for air gone, her grandmother was herself again.

But Jenan is not. One of her pillars is gone, and in that void she's finally found her own strength. "I definitely felt as though I had stepped into a new chapter of my life," she writes when asked about her life after Margaret. "One of uncertainty. I had to become a new person as the one I leaned on, depended on, thrived on was no longer with me. I can't say I felt alone, but independent. …"

Jenan's journey is unlikely to get any easier. Doctors recently found asbestos tracks on her lungs, and though she can't afford the $50 it would take for further testing, she is gearing up to quit smok-ing, promising herself to get more exercise—all the things that might keep her healthier longer. She's falling in love, she tells me, and is making plans to go back to school, to attend the university in Missoula.

"I have finally learned that in any given situation I am not powerless," Jenan writes. She is the keeper of her grandmother's memory, the inheritor of her mother's crusade. "No matter who the Goliath may be, I can be the conqueror," she says. "I am daily learning new lessons. And one day I will step into a new chapter, a new world, and apply them to whatever cause God has laid before me. And this will happen without fear, for I am the successor of the two most courageous women I know."

Gayla says she used to think her job would be finished when the town was clean and safe. Or when the Center for Asbestos Related Disease closed for lack of business. Or when she could have her picture taken putting the "For Sale" sign up outside of Grace's headquarters. Those weren't realistic goals, though she must have needed them to fight so hard for so long. "Now I hope I live long enough to see them do something with the research to literally neutralize this fiber in the body, that within the next twenty years they could come up with something that would make it as harmless as packing a piece of shrapnel in your butt," she says. "That would be good. That's the primary goal now because I know the others are sort of nonsense."

The truth is in her voice: Gayla has found some equilibrium, some peace. The fire that smoldered in her heart as her mother suffocated to death, the flames bursting into an all-consuming rage, is gone. "I don't think the anger is there anymore, the anger I felt when mother was alive," she says. "When I went to court, that was the deal I made with myself. As far as the burning hatred or vendetta, I feel that mother's death has been justified. And that's what she wanted was for people to realize why she was dying. I think she's been more than vindicated at this point.

"Getting this job done and quitting it: it's just something that seemed natural."

There are still fronts on which Libby's battle is being fought: the EPA had to struggle mightily to win the declaration of a public health emergency, which will let them go into people's homes and remove Zonolite insulation.* The Superfund itself is in a precarious position: it may not even exist long enough to finish the cleanup job here. And somehow, everyone in Libby has to make a leap of faith, to trust Paul Peronard enough to tell him where all the hot spots are. If they do, everyone can move on. If they don't, they can never be sure which corners of their town are hiding death from the past. For Libby, everything hangs in that balance.

It is shaping up to be a good mushroom season in Libby's corner of the state: wildfires and heavy snowpack ought to contribute to a decent morel crop. Daily rainstorms have made gardening difficult, but not impossible. As I dump dirt into planters out in front of the house, I recall that the EPA warned recently that bags of Libby vermiculite still sit on the shelves of some stores—asbestos lurking in potting soil and insulation. While things have begun to return to normal in Libby—the camera crews are gone, the EPA has settled into the community like any other storefront operation—what will constitute normal for the foreseeable future is a more cynical reality than existed prior to the autumn of 1999. For the most part the proportions of the nightmare are mapped out, the blame assigned. Court victories helped some citizens with medical bills, but not with the fundamental questions about the loss of innocence and trust.

The river has broken up, the ice floating downstream. Fishing will be good for another month or so, before the snowmelt muddies the water. The maps will come out again, marked by years of creases, in anticipation of finding a new morel mushroom patch or revisiting an old fishing hole. It's always a relief to survive the dark, cold days of a Montana winter, and for those who are sick, each spring is surely a blessing.

---

*That declaration was never made. The implication of such an emergency in Libby would logically apply to the millions of buildings in the rest of the U.S. containing Zonolite insulation. According to a report by Andrew Schneider for the St. Louis Post-Dispatch ("White House blocked EPA's asbestos cleanup plan," 12/29/02), that specter prompted the federal Office of Management and Budget to squash the plan in the spring of 2002. "Instead, Superfund boss [Marianne] Horinko ... quietly ordered that asbestos be removed from contaminated homes in Libby," Schneider reported.

When I call him, Les answers the phone with a strong voice. He's doing really well, he says. He is working on getting a permanent memorial for Libby's asbestos victims built on the courthouse lawn. "Gayla wanted to put it up by Rainy Creek at the entrance to the mine, and I guess that would be okay, but I want to see it downtown where people in town on a day-to-day basis can see it and be reminded of what happened here. So I'm gonna stick for that," he says. "Whether the county will even let us put it on the courthouse lawn is another thing that remains to be seen. If they don't, I'm gonna raise hell with them." The fight is still in him, this frail old man.

The land is full of analogies for life: a forest that endures logging; an old grizzly bear who has learned to survive even as his home valleys are eroded by development; trout that rest in the eddies, feeding just on the edge of the fast water. If there are answers to Libby's questions, they must lie here too—in the mountains that sustained these families even as they tore away at the earth in search of profit, and in the dirt that will bury them all.

Acknowledgments

I'd like to thank everyone from Libby who shared the private details of their lives with me, but I owe an especially large debt to the Benefield and Skramstad families. Their strength and humor inspired and sustained me, and they are directly responsible for any power this book may have.

Many people helped with the research for this project, and more than a few told me they did so for the simple reason that the story needed to be told. The following employees of the Environmental Protection Agency were happy to help whenever I called, some far beyond the call of duty: Paul Peronard, Chris Weis, Duc Nguyen, Linda Newstrom, and Cate Jenkins. Thanks are due to reference librarians Donald Springer of Missoula and Gail Anderson of Libby, to Dave Walter of the Montana State Historical Society, and to the following people who talked with me though it wasn't part of their job description: Roger Sullivan, Allan McGarvey, Andrij Holian, James Lockey, David Egilman, and Richard Irons. I especially appreciate the efforts made by Drs. Alan Whitehouse and Brad Black to make room for me in their very busy schedules. My brother, Michael Barnett, put both his pharmacy and law degrees to good use whenever I called for help with the research, and my good friend Diane Thompson was a quick and astute reader of my early drafts. I also appreciate the professional generosity shown to me by Spokane *Spokesman-Review* reporter Susan Drumheller and Bozeman journalist Todd Wilkinson's candid advice when I was looking for an agent and a publisher.

A number of friends provided desperately needed respite while I was traveling over the past couple of years, and specifically I want to thank Debra Little, Rick Bass, and Mark "Phoenix" Sigalov for their hospitality. The support and encouragement I got from a whole lot of people were crucial to this project, and in particular I owe deepest thanks to my parents, Bob and Diann Barnett; Maryanne Vollers; Terry Tempest-Williams; my editor, Stephen Topping; Johnson Books; and my husband, Doug Peacock.

Bibliography

Abel, Heather. "Montana on the Edge: A Fight over Gold Forces the Treasure State to Confront Its Future." *High Country News* (12/22/97): 1.

Agency for Toxic Substances and Disease Registry. "Mortality from Asbestosis in Libby, Montana." 12/12/00.

———. "Preliminary Findings of Medical Testing of Individuals Potentially Exposed to Asbestoform Minerals Associated with Vermiculite in Libby, Montana." 2/22/01.

———. "Year 2000 Medical Testing of Individuals Potentially Exposed to Asbestoform Minerals Associated with Vermiculite in Libby, Montana." 8/23/01.

Air Hygiene Foundation. Meeting of the Temporary Organization Committee. 2/1/35.

Amandus, H. E., et al. "The Morbidity and Mortality of Vermiculite Miners and Millers Exposed to Tremolite-Actinolite: Part 1. Exposure Estimates." *American Journal of Industrial Medicine* 11 (1987): 1–14.

Ambros, Otto. Letter to Director Dencker. 9/28/44.

———. Memo on professional experience. 11/14/67.

———. Letter to J. Peter Grace. 1/30/80.

American Consulate General. "Request for Records Check." Central Clearance Unit. 4/14/58.

American Society for Testing Materials. Interview with Bradley Dewey. 1936.

Anderson, Ron. Lincoln County Sanitation. "Field Report: Sampling at the Former W.R. Grace Export Plant Site Located on City of Libby Property." 11/16/99–11/17/99.

Application of Montana vermiculite company for decree of dissolution and approval of plan of liquidation. U.S. District Court, Montana, 11th Judicial District, Lincoln County. 7/22/64.

Bank, Walter, and Ronald Uhle. "Health Study (Asbestos Dust): Libby Mine and Mill." Bureau of Mines. Health and Safety Field Group. 5/18/71–5/21/71.

Beagle, Bob. Written testimony for informal panel on proposed Superfund designation. 7/6/01.

Benefield, Gayla. Journal of her mother's death. Undated.

Berger, Elizabeth H. Testimony before the United States Senate Committee on Environment and Public Works: Subcommittee on Clean Air, Wetlands and Climate Change. 2/11/02.

Bjornberg, Victor. "Transcript of Interview with Earl Lovick." Montana Historical Society. Undated.

Bleich, Raymond. Letter to Joseph Kelley. "Senate Bill No. 112, Pertaining to Occupational Diseases in Montana." 4/22/59.

Boal, Pierre de L. Letter to U.S. Secretary of State. "Possible Removal of Dr. Julio Guzman Tellez from Management of W.R. Grace Interests in Bolivia …" 12/18/42.

Bonsal, Philip W. Letter to Woodward (first name unknown). 7/10/42.

Borgstedt, H. Memo to E. S. Wood. "Pleural Effusions." 1/21/79.

Bowditch, Manfred. Letter to Anthony Lanza. 12/10/37.

———. Letter to Bradley Dewey. 2/19/38.

Brodeur, Paul. "The Asbestos Tragedy." In Breath Taken: The Landscape and Biography of Asbestos. Bill Ravanesi, ed. Newtonville, Mass.: Center for Visual Arts in the Public Interest, 1991.

Brown, H. A. Memo to H. C. Duecker and Arnold M. Rosenberg. "Mono-Kote." 3/28/72.

Bruce, David Kirkpatrick. Diary, Volumes 25–35. Kept as U.S. Ambassador to the Federal Republic of Germany. 7/22/58.

Bush, W. M., Jr. Memo to Jack Wolter. "Employee Education and No Smoking Programs—Libby 1977." 4/27/77.

———. Memo to Jack Wolter. "Smoking at Libby." 8/23/76.

Byers, Dohrman. Letter to Benjamin Wake. 9/5/56.

Cairns, James. Letter to Raymond Bleich. 7/20/59.

Cintani, James. Deposition. The Port Authority of New York and New Jersey v. Allied Corporation. U.S. District Court, Southern District of New York. 7/3/96.

Cintani, Jim. Memo to Pete Hollis. "Monthly Situation Report July, 1969." 8/6/69.

———. Memo to Pete Hollis. "Monthly Situation Report September, 1969." 10/3/69.

City of New York. Department of Air Resources. Proclamation regarding asbestos. 4/13/70.

Clayton, Lawrence A. Grace: W.R. Grace & Co., the Formative Years 1850–1930. Ottawa, Ont.: Jameson Books, 1985.

Code of Federal Regulations. "National Emission Standard for Asbestos." Title 40, Ch. 1, Subpart B (7/1/73), pp. 500–506; Federal Register 38(44) (4/6/73): 8820–8822.

Cohea, Teresa Olcott. "Taxation of Metal Mines: A Report to the Forty-Sixth Legislature/Revenue Oversight Committee." Helena: Montana Legislative Council, 1978.

Complaint. United States of America v. W.R. Grace Co.–Conn., Inc. U.S. District Court, District of Montana, Great Falls Division. Undated copy.

"The Confederated Salish and Kootenai Tribes of the Flathead Indian Reservation." Online posting. Char-Koostra News. www.ronan.net (accessed 10/11/01).

Consent decree. United States of America v. W.R. Grace Co.–Conn., Inc. U.S. District Court, District of Montana, Missoula Division. 12/23/94.

Cooke, W. E. "Fibrosis of the Lungs Due to the Inhalation of Asbestos Dust." British Medical Journal (7/25/24): 147.

Culver, William. Letter to "Gentlemen." 5/24/73.

Dally, Michelle. "The Hero Who Wound Up on the Wrong Side of the Law." Rhode Island Monthly (November 2001): 37–105.

Dawson, Allan. Letter to Philip Bonsal. 9/11/42.

Defendant W.R. Grace & Co.–Conn.'s memorandum in opposition to plaintiff's motion to compel responses to plaintiff's discovery. The Ohio Hospital Association v. Armstrong World Industries, Inc. Court of Common Pleas, Cuyahoga County, Ohio. Undated.

Defendant W.R. Grace & Co.–Conn.'s response to plaintiffs' interrogatories and request to supplement prior discovery responses. *The Ohio Hospital Association v. Armstrong World Industries, Inc.* Court of Common Pleas, Cuyahoga County, Ohio. 1/22/98.

Deutsch, Claudia H. "In $5 Billion Deal, Grace Will Sell Packaging Business." *New York Times* (8/15/97): 1D.

Dewey, Bradley. Letter to Manfred Bowditch. 2/23/38.

———. Letter to Henry A. Wallace. 10/23/45.

Dewey, Bradley, Jr. Deposition. *The Port Authority of New York and New Jersey v. Allied Corporation.* U.S. District Court, Southern District of New York. 9/17/96.

Dorfman, Dan. "The Nazi Connection: The Past That Germany's Flick Group and W.R. Grace Won't Talk About." *Esquire* (12/19/78): 14–17.

Dreessen, Waldemar C., et al. "A Study of Asbestosis in the Asbestos Textile Industry." U.S. Public Health Service *Public Health Bulletin No. 241* (8/38): 1–117.

Driscoll, Pat. Letter to Montana Department of Health and Environmental Services. "W.R. Grace Inspection." 5/16/85, 10/15/87.

Dubois, Josiah. *The Devil's Chemists.* Boston: Beacon Press, 1952.

Dugan, C. F. Memo to W. L. Taggart. "Report of Trip to Kalispell, Montana." 12/5/67.

Editorial. "Asbestos Bill Needs Teeth to Serve Victims." Online posting. *Billings Gazette.* www.billingsgazette.com (12/30/99).

Editorial. "Pulmonary Asbestosis." *Journal of the American Medical Association* 95 (1930): 1431.

———. "Asbestosis and Cancer of the Lung." *Journal of the American Medical Association* 140 (8/13/49): 1219–1220.

Edwards, G. H., and J. R. Lynch. "The Method Used by the U.S. Public Health Service for Enumeration of Asbestos Dust on Membrane Filters." *Annals of Occupational Hygiene* 11 (1968): 1–6.

Egan, Thomas. Memo to Regional Managers. 4/9/70.

———. Memo to R. L. Asher et al. 6/1/70.

Egilman, David. Expert Witness Disclosure. *The Port of Authority of New York and New Jersey v. Allied Corporation.* U.S. District Court, Southern District of New York. Undated.

Ellman, P. "Pulmonary Asbestosis: Its Clinical, Radiological, and Pathological Features, and Associated Risk of Tuberculous Infection." *Journal of Industrial Hygiene* 15 (7/33): 165–183.

Environmental Protection Agency. "Public Hearing on National Emissions Standards for Hazardous Air Pollutants." Los Angeles, Calif. 2/15/72–2/16/72.

———. Assessment Division. "Priority Review Level 1—Asbestos-Contaminated Vermiculite." 6/80.

———. Office of Toxic Substances. "Interim Final Report: Exposure Assessment for Asbestos-Contaminated Vermiculite." 2/18/82.

———. Office of Pesticides and Toxic Substances. "Collection, Analysis and Characterization of Vermiculite Samples for Fiber Content and Asbestos Contamination: Final Report." 9/27/82.

———. Chemical Selections and Profiles Team, and Chemical Hazard Identification Branch. "Status Report 8EHQ-0383-0473." 4/20/83.

———. "Inspection Guide and Report: Federal Air Inspection." Region VIII. Inspection date 5/23/89. Report date illegible.

———. "Mining Company Pays Penalty for Clean Air Act Violations." 9/8/94.

———. "EPA Fact Sheet: Asbestos Sampling in Libby, MT." 1/00, 3/00, 5/00.

———. "EPA Fact Sheet: Phase 2 Sampling in Libby, MT." 3/01.

———. "EPA Wins Lawsuit Against Grace and KDC." 3/12/01.

———. "EPA Files Suit Against Grace for Cleanup Costs." 4/2/01.

———. "EPA Fact Sheet: Libby Schools Update." 5/01.

———. "EPA Emergency Responses at World Trade Center and Pentagon." 9/14/01.

———. "EPA, OSHA Update Asbestos Data, Continue to Reassure Public About Contamination Fears." 9/16/01.

———. "Whitman Details Ongoing Agency Efforts to Monitor Disaster Sites, Contribute to Cleanup Efforts." 9/18/01.

———. "Access Lawsuit Settlement Requires W.R. Grace to Provide Community Health Benefits." 10/25/01.

"EPA Agrees to Clinton Call for Air Quality Task Force at Trade Center." Online posting. *Inside EPA* 23(7). www.InsideEpa.com (2/15/02).

Eschenbach, Harry A. Memo to Harry Brown. "Asbestos." 2/10/72.

———. Letter to S. V. Chamberlain. 9/15/78.

———. Memo to Robert Oliverio. "Dr. Irons' Visit." 12/5/78.

———. Memo to Robert Oliverio. "Dr. Irons." 4/10/79.

———. Letter to Richard Irons. 5/8/79.

———. Memo to Jack Wolter. "W.J. McCaig's telephone conversation with Dr. Irons." 7/23/79.

———. Memo to O. Mario Favorito. "EPA Asbestos Inquiry." 1/7/80.

———. Memo to R. C. Ericson. "Inquiry Concerning Vermiculite." 5/20/82.

———. Memo to V. Bakeman et al. "Mortality Study—Richard Monson." 7/28/82.

———. Letter to EPA Document Control Officer. 3/24/83.

———. Memo to J. Berke et al. "Libby Study/NIOSH." 10/4/83.

———. Memo to R. C. Walsh. "Meeting 17 October 1983, Patrick Sebastien and Ben Armstrong." 10/18/83.

———. Memo to E. S. Wood. "Libby X-ray History." 4/21/81.

———. Deposition. *Ervin E. Hurlbert, et al. v. W.R. Grace & Co.* U.S. District Court, Montana, 19th Judicial District, Lincoln County. 4/1/97.

———. Testimony. *T.H.S. Northstar Association v. W.R. Grace & Co., et al.* U.S. District Court, District of Minnesota, Third Division. 11/16/93.

"Excerpts from Farben-Auschwitz Weekly Report No. 11 for the Period 3–9 August 1941." Prosecution Exhibit 1985. *Trials of War Criminals before the Nuremberg Military Tribunals*, Vol. VIII, Washington, D.C.: United States Printing Office, 1952.

"Fairness in Asbestos Compensation Act of 1998." U.S. Senate Bill 758, 105th/106th Congress.

Farner, Lloyd W. Letter to John Meyer. 9/22/41.

———. Letter to John Meyer. 2/11/42.

Favorito, Mario. Letter to Daniel Banks. 2/11/81.

———. Letter to Thomas J. Shepich. "Proposed NIOSH Vermiculite Study." 6/29/81.

Federal Bureau of Investigation. "German Activity Among Coffee Fincas in Guatemala." 5/16/42.

Feit, Thomas. Memo to Bruce R. Williams. "Environmental Protection Agency Proposed Standards for Air Emissions of Asbestos." 6/8/72.

Flint, Myles E., and Sara D. Himmelhoch. Letter to Bill Robinson. "United States v. W.R. Grace & Co.–Conn., Inc." 2/8/93.

"Former Montana Governor Marc Racicot—Biography." Online posting. *Discovering Montana*. www.discoveringmontana.com (accessed 2/14/02).

"Fortune 500 List." *Fortune*. 1955–2000.

Gardner, Dr. Leroy U. Letter to Anthony Lanza. 12/14/37.

———. Letter to Manfred Bowditch. 3/22/38.

———. Letter to J. P. Woodard, 5/8/46.

Geiger, Randy. Memo to Robert Oliverio. "Requested Data for Forthcoming Visits of Management." 6/30/77.

———. Memo to William McCaig. "High School Track Air Samples." 7/8/81.

Gloyne, S. R. "The Morbid Anatomy and Histology of Asbestosis." *Tubercle* 14 (9/33): 550–558.

Gordon, George. Letter to Adolph A. Berle, Jr. 5/2/41.

Grace Bankruptcy News. *Bankruptcy Creditors Service, Inc.* 1 (4/3/01): 1–14.

Graf, Carl N. Deposition. *The Port of Authority of New York and New Jersey v. Allied Corporation*. U.S. District Court, Southern District of New York. 9/20/96.

Grandstaff, Carlotta. "To Be or Not to Be?" Online posting. *Missoula Independent*. www.missoulanews.com (7/19/01).

Granger, Hugh, et al. "Preliminary Health Hazard Assessment: World Trade Center." 10/2/01.

Guillemot, Fred. Memo to Dick Aishton. "Zonolite R-4339, Tampa, Florida." 4/5/72.

Guthrie, Andrea. Memo to Amy Taylor. "W.R. Grace Vermiculite Mine, Libby MT." 3/4/92.

Hill, Ted. Memo to Larry Lloyd. "Trip Report—Libby (W.R. Grace, Co.)—Feb. 4–8, 1974." 2/11/74.

———. Letter to Robert Oliverio. 6/10/74.

Himmelhoch, Sarah. Letter to Andrea Guthrie and Shelly Cleverly. 2/8/94.

Hintze, Lynnette. "W.R. Grace Penalized for Closing Gates." Online posting. *Daily Inter Lake Newspaper*. www.dailyinterlake.com (10/26/01).

Holiday, Bob. "Added Stories of Zonolite History." Lincoln County Public Library. Undated.

Hooper, William A. Letter to Kathleen Kennedy. 4/9/80.

———. Letter to David Robinson. 5/2/80.

————. Letter to Warren Norton. 12/7/84.

Hoover, J. Edgar. Memo to Adolph A. Berle, Jr. "Surveillance of Floyd E. Nelson in Lima, Peru, from April 30, 1942 to May 7, 1942." 7/21/42.

————. Memo to Adolph A. Berle, Jr. "Floyd E. Nelson, Panagra Pilot." Undated.

Howard, Joseph Kinsey. *Montana: High, Wide and Handsome*. Lincoln: University of Nebraska Press, 1983.

Hunt, Linda. *Secret Agenda: The United States Government, Nazi Scientists, and Project Paperclip, 1945–1990*. New York: St. Martin's Press, 1991.

Industrial Hygiene Foundation. "Research." 11/10/42.

————. Members of the Industrial Hygiene Foundation. 1943.

Intelligence Department of the Army, from the Assistant Chief of Staff. "Dossier No. XEO21877. Ambrose, Otto." 6/29/73.

Interagency "for your information" note to Montana EPA director John Wardell on "'Vermiculite' as an Emerging Chemical Problem." 11/9/84.

Irons, Richard. Letter to Earl Lovick. 3/19/79.

————. Letter to Harry Eschenbach. 4/3/79.

James, Marquis. *Merchant Adventurer: The Story of W.R. Grace*. Wilmington, Del.: Scholarly Resources Inc., 1993.

Jannot, Mark. "The Further Explorations of Piotr Chmielinski." *National Geographic Adventure* (January/February 2002): 41–49.

Jenkins, Cate. Memo to Affected Parties and Responsible Officials. 12/3/01, 12/19/01, 1/11/02, 3/11/02.

————. Memo to Affected Parties and Responsible Officials. "NYC Department of Health Misrepresentations." 2/10/02.

Johns-Manville Corporation. "Asbestos and Health Presentations." 12/7/73.

Johnson, William. Letter to Benjamin Wake. 11/2/71.

"Judge Orders W.R. Grace to Give EPA Access to Montana Property for Cleanup." Online posting. *Chemical Regulation Daily*. www.bna.com/products/ens/crdm.htm (3/14/01).

Keenan, Robert. Letter to Benjamin Wake. 4/13/62.

Kelley, Joseph. Letter to George Blackwood. 1/13/65.

Kennedy, John. Letter to Charles Auer and Hays Bell. 12/5/78.

Kennedy, Kathleen. Letter to Larry Lloyd. 3/19/80.

Knight, A. C. Letter to Earl Lovick. 3/10/59.

"Kootenai Falls: A River Runs over It." Online posting. *KooteNet*. www.libby.org (accessed 10/11/01).

Kostic, Peter. Memo to John F. Murphy. "Zonolite Dust Conditions." 3/29/66.

————. Memo to Harry Brown. "Meeting with Representatives of Bureau of Mines, Denver." 12/17/71.

"Kutenai Indians." *Nelson BC*. www.nelsonbc.ca (accessed 10/11/01).

Lanza, A. J., W. J. McConnell, and J. W. Fehnel. "Effects of the Inhalation of Asbestos Dust on the Lungs of Asbestos Workers." Oxford University Press: *Public Health Reports* 50 (1/4/35): 1–12.

Larrick, S. Y. Memo to John Hopkins. "Claim of Lilas D. Welch." 11/25/67.

Levine, Louis. *The Taxation of Mines in Montana*. New York: B.W. Huebsch, 1919.

Levine, Mark. "Killing Libby." *Men's Journal* (8/01): 77–94.

Little, William, M.D. Deposition. *Gayla I. Benefield, et al. v. W.R. Grace & Co.–Conn.* U.S. District Court, Montana, 19th Judicial District, Lincoln County. 7/22/97.

Locke, R. H. Memo to Mario Favorito. "NIOSH Meeting: November 4, 1980." 11/26/80.

Lockey, J. E., et al. "Pulmonary Changes After Exposure to Vermiculite Contaminated with Fibrous Tremolite." *American Review of Respiratory Diseases* 129 (1984): 952–958.

"Loose Asbestos Fiber Seen as Cancer Threat to Men in Building Trades." *Engineering News Record* (4/2/70): 11–12.

Lovick, E. D. Letter to A. C. Knight. 4/1/59.

———. Letter to C. A. Pratt. 6/14/61.

———. Memo to Robert Oliverio. "1978 Chest X-Rays." 12/5/78.

———. Memo to Robert Oliverio. "Dr. Little's X-Ray Classifications." 1/16/79.

———. Memo to Harry Eschenbach. "Proposed Epidemiological Study Protocol." 9/30/81.

———. "Zonolite: A Brief History of the Libby Operation." Lecture notes, Lincoln County Public Library. Undated.

Lovick, Earl D. Deposition. *Ervin E. Hurlbert, et al. v. W.R. Grace & Co.* U.S. District Court, Montana, 19th Judicial District, Lincoln County. 12/19/96, 4/3/97, 4/4/97, 4/16/97.

Lynch, Jeremiah R. Letter to Benjamin Wake. 10/17/68.

Lynch, Jeremiah. Deposition. *Finstad v. W.R. Grace & Co.* U.S. District Court, Montana, 19th Judicial District, Lincoln County. 4/13/99.

Lynch, K. M., and Atmar W. Smith. "Asbestosis Bodies in Sputum and Lung." *Journal of the American Medical Association* 95 (8/30/30): 659–661.

Malone, Michael. *Montana: A Contemporary Profile.* Helena: Farcountry Press, 1996.

Malter, Martin. Letter to C. Weber. 7/20/67.

McCaig, Bill. Memo to Jack Wolter. "Telephone Conversation with Dr. Richard Irons Held 3:30 PM on July 3 Concerning Our Medical Surveillance Program." 7/5/79.

———. Memo to Jack Wolter. "James L. Gidley, Deceased." 1/25/83.

———. Memo to Jack Wolter. "Mandatory Showers and Uniform Policy for Libby Employees." 7/15/83.

———. Letter to Bob Raisch. 2/24/84.

———. Memo to Jack Wolter. "Inquiry Concerning Health of Libby Operation Employees." 5/6/85.

McCaig, William. Deposition. *Ervin E. Hurlbert, et al. v. W.R. Grace & Co.* U.S. District Court, Montana, 19th Judicial District, Lincoln County. 3/25/97.

McDonald, Howard. Letter to Editor. *Coeur d'Alene Press.* 6/8/01.

McDonald, J. C., et al. "Cohort Study of Mortality of Vermiculite Miners Exposed to Tremolite." *British Journal of Industrial Medicine* 43 (1986): 436–444.

McGrath, Mike. Letter to Judy Martz. "Libby/W.R. Grace." 8/13/01.

———. Memo to Judy Martz. "W.R. Grace & Co.'s Cleanup of Asbestos Contamination at Libby." 8/13/01.

McKague, J. V. Memo to Harry Brown. "Zonolite—Stack Emissions, Winnipeg." 11/16/71.

Mellon Institute of Industrial Research. "Symposium on Dust Problems." 1/15/35.

Memo (unsigned) to Montana Governor Ted Schwinden, outlining issues for impending visit with Grace's Bill McCaig. 9/26/85.

Merchant, James A. Letter to Thomas J. Shepich. 4/27/81.

Merewether, E. R. A., and C. W. Price. *Report on Effects of Asbestos Dust on the Lungs and Dust Suppression in the Asbestos Industry.* London: H.M. Stationery Office, 1930.

Military Attaché Report. "Subversive Activities—Oruro." Military Intelligence Division, War Department General Staff. Report 132a. 1/26/42.

Moatamed, Farhad, James A. Lockey, and William T. Parry. "Fiber Contamination of Vermiculites: A Potential Occupational and Environmental Health Hazard." *Environmental Research* 41 (1986): 207–218.

Molloy, Donald W., Judge. Order. *United States of America v. W.R. Grace & Co. and Kootenai Development Corporation.* U.S. District Court, District of Montana. 3/9/01.

Monson, Richard R. "Cause of Death Among Sixty-six Libby Employees." Harvard School of Public Health. 4/5/82.

Montana Code Annotated. "Industrial Hygiene." Session Laws of the 40th Legislative Assembly. Ch. 197, S. 19-23, pp. 474–475. 1959.

Montana Department of Commerce. "Montana County Statistical Report: Lincoln County." Census and Economic Information Center. 1996.

Montana Department of Environmental Quality. "Final Environmental Assessment for Dillon Vermiculite Application for Operating Permit." 4/16/99.

———. "Libby Asbestos Investigation: DEQ Updates." 12/14/99, 12/15/99.

———. "Libby Update." 10/16/00.

———. "W.R. Grace File Review Summary: Chronological Order of Events (CVID #3726)." Undated.

Montana Department of State Lands. "Draft Environmental Assessment for W.R. Grace Vermiculite Closure Plan near Libby, MT." Hard Rock Bureau. 8/19/92.

Montana Historical Society and U.S. Army Corps of Engineers. "The Search for the Kootenai Past: A Seminar on the Kootenai Region of the United States and Canada." 8/3/79–8/4/79.

"Montana Enviros Hit Burns on Asbestos." Online posting. *National Journal Group.* www.nationaljournal.com (1/24/00).

Montana Supreme Court. Opinion in the case of *Louise N. Gidley v. W.R. Grace & Company.* 4/15/86.

Moran, Mike. Letter to Harry Eschenbach. "OSHA's Label Requirement on MK-3." 3/30/73.

Moss, Michael, and Adrianne Appel. "Protecting the Product: Company's Silence Countered Safety Fears About Asbestos." Online posting. *New York Times.* www.nytimes.com (7/9/01).

Nance, James W. "Congressional Inquiry Regarding the Appointment of J. Peter Grace." Memorandum for the White House. 3/23/82.

———. Letter to Tom Lantos. 4/13/82.

Nelson, Woodrow. Letter to Joseph Kelley. 8/25/64.

"New Specifications Eliminate Asbestos [illegible] Trade Center." *Newark Evening News* (5/28/70): 29.

Norweb, Henry R. Letter to Secretary of State. "Certain Employees on Board Grace Line Vessels with Reported Axis Leanings." 1/15/42.

Nystrong, Markus. "Witness Testimony: Professor David Egilman Fights the Asbestos Industry." Online posting. *College Hill Independent.* www.netspace.org/~indy/issues/4.8.99/current/news3.html (accessed 10/4/01).

O'Keefe, Mark. Legal Memorandum re: U.S. Senate Bill 758. 1/21/00.

Oliverio, Robert. Memo to Jack Wolter. "Health Problems—Salaried Personnel." 12/4/78.

Oulton, Stacie. "Expert's Testimony in Flats Suit Stricken." Online posting. *Denver Post.* www.denverpost.com (6/19/01).

Pardee, J. T., and E. S. Larsen. "Deposits of Vermiculite and Other Minerals in the Rainy Creek District, near Libby, Montana." In *Contributions to Economic Geology, Part 1: Metals and Nonmetals Except Fuels.* G. F. Loughlin and G. R. Mansfield, geologists in charge. Washington, D.C.: U.S. Geological Survey, 1929.

Parloff, Roger. "The $200 Billion Miscarriage of Justice." Online posting. *Fortune.* www.fortune.com (3/4/02).

Pickthall, Walt. Memo to Fred Eaton. "Bay Area Air Pollution Control." 8/6/71.

Platenberg, Patrick. Montana Department of Health and Environmental Services. "W.R. Grace Inspection." 12/10/87.

Raisch, Bob. Letter to Earl Lovick. 1/31/84.

Robinson, Dave. Letter to H. M. Dixon. Undated.

Rogers, William. Letter to John Doe. 4/2/71.

Rosenberg, Arnold M. Deposition. *Anchorage School District v. W.R. Grace & Co.* U.S. District Court, District of Alaska. 5/19/87.

Schepers, Gerrit. "Chronology of Asbestos Cancer Discoveries: Experimental Studies of the Saranac Laboratory." *American Journal of Industrial Medicine* 27 (1995): 593–606.

Schneider, Andrew. "Uncivil Action." *Seattle Post-Intelligencer.* Series. 11/18/99–11/19/99.

———. "White House blocked EPA's asbestos cleanup plan." *St. Louis Post-Dispatch.* 12/29/02.

Seelye, Katharine Q. "Bush Proposing to Shift Burden of Toxic Cleanup to Taxpayers." Online posting. *New York Times.* www.nytimes.com (2/24/02).

Selikoff, Irving J., Jacob Churg, and Cuyler E. Hammond. "Asbestos Exposure and Neoplasia." *Journal of the American Medical Association* 188 (4/6/64): 22–26.

Selikoff, Irving J., Cuyler E. Hammond, and Jacob Churg. "Asbestos Exposure, Smoking and Neoplasia." *Journal of the American Medical Association* 204 (4/8/68): 104–110.

Simonich, Mark. "Field Hearing in Libby, MT." Report to the U.S. Senate Committee on Environment and Public Works. 2/16/00.

Skramstad, Lester. Deposition. *Lester Skramstad and Norita Skramstad v. W.R. Grace & Co.* U.S. District Court, Montana, 19th Judicial District, Lincoln County. 1/13/97.

Smith, William E. "Biologic Tests of Tremolite in Hamsters." Presented to the Society for Occupational and Environmental Health. 12/6/77.

———. "Final Report on Biologic Tests of Samples 22260p5 and 22263p2." Health Research Institute, Fairleigh Dickinson University. 5/25/78.

"Sprayed-Asbestos Fireproofing Work Halted." *Engineering News-Record* (5/7/70): 21.

Springer, Donald. *Waters of Wealth: The Story of the Kootenai River and Libby Dam.* Boulder: Pruett Publishing Co., 1979.

Stewart, M. J., N. Tattersall, and A. C. Haddow. "On the Occurrence of Clumps of Asbestosis Bodies in the Sputum of Asbestos Workers." *Journal of Pathology* 35 (1932): 737–741.

Stockholm International Peace Research Institute. "Sarin." Online posting. *Chemical and Biological Warfare Project.* www.projects.sipri.se/cbw/cbwagents/Sarin.html (accessed 3/17/02).

Stringer, Alan. "If More Was Needed, Grace, EPA Equally Responsible." Online posting. *Western News.* www.thewesternnews.com (8/22/01).

Thomson, Robert D. Deposition. *Robert D. Thomson v. W.R. Grace & Co.* Montana, 4th Judicial District Court, Missoula County. 4/20/88.

Tilley, Major E. Letter to P. M. Wilson. 11/7/45.

Transcript of Proceedings. *Lester Skramstad and Norita Skramstad v. W.R. Grace & Co.* U.S. District Court, Montana, 19th Judicial District, Lincoln County. 5/19/97–5/20/97.

U.S. Control Group Council. Memorandum on Dr. Otto Ambrose. Office of the Director of Intelligence, Field Information Agency to the Assistant Chief of Staff, United States Forces, European Theater. 9/13/45.

U.S. Department of Labor. "Evaluation of MSHA's Handling of Inspections at the W.R. Grace & Company Mine in Libby, Montana." Office of Inspector General. 3/22/01.

———. "EPA's Actions Concerning Asbestos-Contaminated Vermiculite in Libby, Montana." Office of Inspector General. 3/31/01.

U.S. Department of State. Telegram to U.S. Embassy, Lima, Peru. 5/27/41.

U.S. Embassy, La Paz, Bolivia. "Activities of Colonel Meliton Brito and Dr. Hans Kemski." Confidential Dispatch no. 513 to U.S. Secretary of State. 8/21/42.

———. "Activities of Colonel Meliton Brito." Confidential Dispatch no. 485 to U.S. Secretary of State. 8/23/42.

U.S. Secretary of State. Request for comment from U.S. Embassy in La Paz regarding Col. Meliton Brito. 8/6/42.

Veltman, P. L. Letter to J. G. Mark. 2/1/63.

"Vermiculite Asbestos." Unsigned memo to J. Peter Grace. 10/1/76.

Vining, R. M. Memo to William Copulsky. "Sprayed Fire Retardants." 4/10/70.

Wake, Benjamin. Letter to Dohrman Byers. 8/13/56.

———. Montana State Board of Health. "A Report on an Industrial Hygiene Study of the Zonolite Company of Libby, Montana." 9/21/56, 112/59, 4/19/62, 4/11/63.

———. Letter to Robert Keenan. 3/13/62.

———. Letter to Raymond Bleich. 7/3/63.

———. Letter to Arthur Bundrock. 4/13/64.

———. Inspection report of Grace facilities. 5/11/64.

———. Letter to Raymond Bleich. 10/2/64.

Walter, Dave. "A Brief History of Lincoln County, Montana." Montana Historical Society. 2/80.

Walworth, Herbert. Letter to John Meyer. 10/11/41.

War Crimes Office. "File No. 86-2-1-BK-1 Farben." Judge Advocate General's
Office. Undated.

Washington Department of Labor and Industries. "Informal Conference: Zonolite, Division of W.R. Grace & Company." 12/19/73.

Wedler, H. W. "Lung Cancer in Asbestosis Patients." Heidelberg Open Clinic,
Deutsches Archiv fur Klinische Medizin. (1943): 189–209.

Western News. Various articles. 1923–2002.

Whitehouse, Alan C., Dr. Testimony. *Lester Skramstad and Norita Skramstad v.
W.R. Grace & Co.* U.S. District Court, Montana, 19th Judicial District, Lincoln County. 5/15/97.

———. Draft comments for congressional hearing on Libby. 7/26/01.

Whitman, Christine Todd. Letter to Jerrold Nadler. Undated.

Wietelman, Ron. Memo to all Scott employees. 5/20/76.

Williams, Bruce R. Letter to Robert Sansom. 6/14/72.

———. Letter to Robert Sansom. 7/7/72.

———. Letter to E. S. Wood. "Policy Position on Statements Regarding Tremolite in Monokote, Zonolite 330 and Mine Sealant." 3/31/77.

Williams, Bruce R., and Thomas P. Feit. Letter to Dale Slaughter. 5/26/72.

Wilson, Edward D. Memo to Fred Fielding. "Nance Correspondence with Rep.
Lantos." 4/15/82.

Wolter, Jack W. Memo to E. S. Wood. "Subject: Libby High School Track Air
Samples." 7/27/81.

Wood, E. S. Memo to W. R. Hanlon et al. "Guidelines for Handling of Tremolite
Contamination in Our Mines, Plants and Products." 3/28/77.

———. Memo to Tremolite File. "Professional Epidemiological Study of Employees Exposed to Tremolite Fibers." 4/21/77.

———. Memo to C. E. Brookes and Carl Graf. "Tremolite in Vermiculite." 5/24/77.

———. Memo to Jack Wolter. "OSHA Citations for MacArthur Company."
5/17/78.

Wood, W. B., and S. R. Gloyne. "Pulmonary Asbestosis: A Review of One Hundred Cases." *The Lancet* (12/22/34): 1383–1385.

"Workers Dead from Asbestos Disease." Exhibit 225, based on death certificates
evaluated by Dr. Alan Whitehouse. Used in multiple cases by McGarvey,
Heberling, Sullivan & McGarvey (law firm), Kalispell, Mont.

W.R. Grace & Co. "Acquisition of Zonolite Company." Report. RCA 225. 1962.

———. "Study of the Interior Fire Protection Requirements of the Exterior
Columns for the World Trade Center Project." Prepared by Martin Malter. 4/8/68.

———. "Study to Determine Relationship Between Years of Employment, Age,
Smoking Habits and Chest X-Ray Findings, Zonolite/Libby Employees." 1969.

———. "Insitu and Environmental Dust Controls for Vermiculite Mining and
Expanding Operations." Report prepared by Fred Eaton, Ray Kujawa, and
Peter Kostic. 3/3/69.

————. "Zonolite Vermiculite Ore Review." Prepared by Harry Brown and O. Floyd Stewart. 7/24/69.

————. Consolidated Monthly Summaries. June–September 1970, December 1970, January 1971.

————. "Performance Report: U.S. Zonolite Operations." 4/3/75.

————. "Fiber Level Reductions." Report. 1977.

————. "Employee Education and No Smoking Program—Libby 1977." Proposed program. 4/27/77.

————. "Dust Control Projects—Libby." List. 4/11/77.

————. "Zonolite Study—Financial Impact of Contingency Plans." 5/6/77.

————. "Tremolite." Presentation to supervisors. 1/19/78.

————. "What You Should Know About Tremolite and Health." Brochure. 1/19/78.

————. "Employee Tremolite Education and No Smoking Program for Libby 1977–1978." Timeline. 2/20/78.

————. "Projected Problems and Costs to Meet Proposed 1.0 and 0.5 Fiber Standards at Libby." Memo prepared by Randy Geiger. 8/11/78.

————. "Minutes of the meeting held with the Union Executive Committee and Company representatives." Prepared by Earl Lovick. 3/21/79.

————. "Occupational Health Report." 5/15/79–5/16/79.

————. "Tremolite—No-Smoking Program." Transcript. 6/1/79.

————. "Employee Tremolite Education and No Smoking Program May 1979." Outline of presentation to employees. 6/8/79.

————. "Air Pollution Improvements." List prepared by Earl Lovick. 7/24/79.

————. "Environmental Data." Response to NIOSH inquiry. 11/18/80.

————. "Facility Audit Draft Report: Zonolite—Libby." 6/81.

————. Comments submitted in response to OSHA proposed rulemaking. 5/24/84.

————. "Air Pollution Abatement—Capital Costs." List. 10/10/84.

————. "Review of Grace's Action Program on the Legislative, Regulatory and Public Awareness Environment Surrounding the Issue of Asbestos-Containing Materials in Buildings." 2/7/86.

————. "Grace to Merge Cryovac Business with Sealed Air in Tax-Free Transaction Creating Two New Public Companies." Press release. 8/14/97.

————. "Grace Urges State of Montana and U.S. EPA to Move Quickly to Address Reported Health Concerns in Libby, Montana." Press release. 11/22/99.

————. "Grace CEO Meets with Montana Governor: Pledges Cooperation on Libby Investigations." Press release. 12/1/99.

————. Annual Reports. 1999, 2000.

————. "Grace Announces Sweeping Health Care Program for Libby, Montana, Residents." Press release. 1/20/00.

————. "Grace Pleased with Decision on Montana Property Rights." Press release. 1/11/01.

————. "Fireproof Material." Table 6. Breakdown of ingredients in Monokote. Undated.

Index

Abel, Heather: on mining industry, 126
Absaroka-Beartooth Wilderness, Noranda and, 130
"Acquisition of Zonolite Company," 62
Addison, John: on asbestos, 196
AFL-CIO, 134, 150
Agency for Toxic Substances and Disease Registry, 207
Agent Orange, 49
AHERA. See Asbestos Hazard Emergency Response Act
Air Hygiene Foundation, 158
Air quality, 81, 144, 146, 158
  indoor, 157
  monitoring, 169
  standards, 132, 133–34
Algonkian Belt series, 30
Alley, Edward, 30, 62
  death of, 34
  enterprise of, 32, 33
  home of, 20–21
  vermiculite and, 31
All Things Considered, 201
Ambrose, Otto, 56–57
  Buna and, 63
  conviction of/sentence for, 58–59, 61
  Grace and, 59, 60–61, 62
American Conference on Governmental Hygienists, 135
American Industrial Association, 176
American Journal of Industrial Medicine, 160
American Legion hall, town meeting at, 216
AmeriCares, 52
Amine, 48
Anaconda Copper Mining Company, 125, 126, 128, 129, 131
Antibiotics, 14
ARCO. See Atlantic Richfield Company
A River Runs Through It (Maclean), 130
Armour, Lester, 34
Armour, Phillip, 34
Armour Meat Packing Company, 34
Aryan Nations, 24
ASARCO, Cabinet-Yaak Wilderness and, 130
Asbestiforms, 139
Asbestos
  amphibole, 30, 120
  analyzing, 170
  blue, 120

breathing, 98, 155
classification of, 86, 87
commercial, 36, 37, 101, 118
controlling, 132, 150
danger of, 90, 162
detecting, 168
emissions of, 133
fibrosis and, 100, 119
forms of, 106
geology of, 97
impact of, 25–26, 38, 96, 209
levels of, 75, 83–84, 172, 173
removing, 177
separation of, 48
serpentine, 120
spray-on, 164, 177
tramp, 60, 145
white, 120
Asbestos fibers, 47, 67, 75, 97, 113–14, 120, 144, 168, 171
  detectable, 172
  doses of, 114, 136
  politics/controversy over, 172
  protection against, 179
  questions about, 100, 115
Asbestos Hazard Emergency Response Act (AHERA), 171, 172
Asbestosis, 9, 13, 77, 96, 100–101, 103, 112, 114, 179, 205
  cancer and, 100, 161
  children and, 180
  compensation for, 81–82
  diagnosis of, 6, 10, 49, 98–99, 152, 184
  effects of, 16–17, 181
  heart problems and, 97
  impact of, 95
  incidence of, 159, 173
  latency period for, 149
  nonminers and, 149
  silicosis and, 97
  testimony on, 115
  winter and, 46–47
Asbestos problem, 74, 83, 119, 122, 134, 198
  EPA and, 146
  government and, 151
  publicity about, 202–3
Asbestos project, 41, 86
Asbestos-related disease, 9–10, 12, 13, 67, 77, 78, 90, 112–13, 117, 121, 137, 163
  answers about, 124
  deaths from, 64
  diagnosis with, 38, 119, 183, 207, 212
  health agencies and, 118

nonoccupational, 149
testing for, 207
understanding, 104
Asbestos School Hazard Detection and Control Act, 172
Asthma, 113, 114, 119, 120
Atlantic Richfield Company (ARCO), 126–27
Auschwitz, 57, 60, 61
Autoimmune disease, 119, 120

Baker, Walter, 74
Ball fields, 69–70, 213
  cleaning up, 208
  contaminated, 189, 193, 207, 214, 215
  Zonolite and, 35
Bank of China Tower, Grace and, 169
Bankruptcy, 49, 51, 127, 179, 181, 207, 213, 217
  victims and, 210
Bankruptcy's Creditor Service, 210
Banks, Dr., 142, 143
Barnett, Clarence: on Guzman Tellez, 55–56
Benefield, David, 7, 8, 19, 155, 188
Benefield, Gayla Vatland
  anger of, 185
  on asbestosis, 13, 99
  criticism of, 155, 198, 202
  on Dale, 8
  described, 3, 5
  Dillon and, 196, 197
  on Egilman, 53
  Eva and, 4, 6
  on father, 5
  on genetic research, 119
  lawsuit by, 185, 187–88
  Les and, 46, 67, 183, 184
  Libby story and, 182
  library of, 193, 200
  Martz and, 155, 217
  medical expenses and, 18
  meeting, 186
  memorial and, 222
  mother and, 5, 7, 10, 12, 14–19
  Norita and, 28
  party for, 154
  richness of, 189, 190
  settlement and, 187, 188, 189
  town meeting and, 216
Benefield, Stacey, 1, 2, 13, 186
Berger, Elizabeth: testimony of, 156–57
Berkeley Pit, 127
Berkeley Square, Grace and, 169

237

Big Blackfoot, 130
Big Mountain, 100
Bin Laden, Osama, 157
Bison, controversy over,
    147–48
Black, Brad, 96, 103, 105
    on asbestos-related disease,
    78, 104
    CARD and, 95
    Irons and, 111
    on medical coverage, 207
    White Lung program and,
    115
Black Mica and Micalite
    Companies, 33
Blaylock, Chuck, 147
Bleich, Raymond "Butch," 74,
    184, 186
    death of, 77
    5 count and, 70
Boeck, Amy, 16, 201
Boston Department of Labor, 63
Breathing apparatuses, 170,
    175
Breathing tests, 78
Brink, Henry, 30
British Journal of Industrial
    Medicine, 141
Brito, Meliton, 55
Broncho-Saline, 14, 18
Brooks, Stuart, 138–39
Brown, Hyman: on Monokote,
    164, 166
Brown, Vandiver, 162
Bruce, David Kirkpatrick, 59
Brus, Roger, 103
Buna, 58, 63
Bundrock, Art, 152, 153
Bundrock, Bill, 152
Bundrock, Helen, 153, 189,
    216
    on anger, 152
    settlement for, 185
Bundrock, Ryan, 153
    asbestosis for, 152
Burlington Northern railroad,
    69, 72
Burnett, Judy, 213
Burnett, Mel, 213
Burns, Conrad, 122
Bush, George W., 199
    Racicot and, 124, 147
Business community, 204,
    214–15
Butte, battles in, 125, 131

Cabinet-Yaak Wilderness,
    ASARCO and, 130
Cairns, James, 101–2
Cancer, 171, 174
    asbestos and, 99, 100,
    159–63, 172, 173
    asbestosis and, 100, 161
    cervical, 12
    chrysotile and, 161
    tremolite and, 109
    See also Lung cancer

Canyon Resources, 130
CARD. See Center for
    Asbestos Related Diseases
Caregiving, 16
Carnegie, Andrew, 51
Carney Creek, waste in, 36, 40
Casa Grace, 51
CBS Laboratories, 62
Center for Asbestos Related
    Diseases (CARD), 78,
    95–96, 220
Center for Environmental
    Health Sciences, 116
Chaloupka, Bill, 130
Chamber of Commerce
    Darko and, 129
    frustrations of, 203, 214
    Lovick and, 35
    Martz and, 198, 216–17
    Peronard and, 72
    Spence and, 149
Charlemagne, 96
Chase Manhattan Bank, Grace
    and, 212
Chisholm, Curt, 129, 130
Chmielinski, Piotr, 177
    on airborne fibers, 178, 179
    TEM and, 176
    WTC and, 171–72
Chronic obstructive
    pulmonary disease
    (COPD), 9
"Chronology of Asbestos
    Cancer Discoveries:
    Experimental Studies of
    the Saranac Laboratory"
    (Schepers), 160
Chrysotile, 63, 64, 120, 141,
    145, 164, 174, 176
    cancer and, 161, 162
    inhalation of, 160
    Monokote-3 and, 166
Cintani, Jim: on Monokote,
    165
City Centre, Grace and, 169
City of New York, 166
    asbestos-containing
    materials and, 165
Civil Action, A (Schlichtman),
    184
Clark, William, 23, 125
Claustrophobia, asbestosis and,
    16–17
Clayton, Lawrence, 51, 52
Cleanup, 72–73, 199, 201,
    207–8, 212
    funds for, 198, 213
    Grace and, 208
Cleveland, Grover, 51
Coal severance tax (1975),
    127
Cohea, Teresa Olcott, 128
Cohenour, Bob, 41, 42
Cole, Floyd: lung disease for,
    77
Commercial Club, Alley and,
    33

Consumer Products Safety
    Council (CPSC), 163
COPD. See Chronic
    obstructive pulmonary
    disease
Copper mining, 86, 125–27
Corcoran, William, 164, 206
Costello, Albert J., 181, 211
Crane, Dan, 173, 174–75
Craver, Tom: death of, 79, 80
Crocidolite, 120
Cryovac, 59, 211
Culver, William: Monokote-3
    and, 167

Daly, Marcus, 125
Darko, Paula, 128, 129
Dateline, 201
Davison Chemical Company,
    51, 159
Dawson, Allen, 55
Death benefits, 182
Death certificates, 135, 206
Dedrick, Bob, 121, 122, 123,
    154
Dedrick, Carrie, 121, 122, 123,
    154
Dement, John, 140
Department of Environmental
    Quality (DEQ), 122, 192
    criticism of, 129
    Dillon and, 195–96
    mine expansion proposal
    and, 195
    Stansbury and, 194, 196
Department of Health, 132, 133
Department of Labor, 141
Department of Mines, 162
DEQ. See Department of
    Environmental Quality
DeShazer, Jack, Jr., 204
    on publicity, 202–3
    on real estate market, 203
DeShazer, Jack, Sr., 218, 219
DeShazer, Tom: lung disease
    for, 77
Devil's Chemists, The (DuBois),
    58
Dewey, Bradley, Jr., 59, 61
Dewey, Bradley, Sr., 63
Dewey and Almy Chemical
    Company, 51, 59, 63
Dillon, vermiculite mine at,
    194–97
Disaster sites, 169–70
Discovery Channel, 201
Doll, Richard: on lung cancer,
    99
Dolliver, Richard, 83
Dow Chemical, Ambrose and,
    62
Dreessen, Waldemar, 75, 159,
    175
Driscoll, Pat, 132, 133, 134
Dry mill, 37, 39, 40, 48, 76, 83
    asbestos content of, 70
    closing, 81, 98, 180

dust in, 76, 80
working in, 67, 82
DuBois, Josiah: on Ambrose, 58
Dugan, Charles, 82
Dust, 36, 37, 40, 47, 62, 86, 156, 179, 196, 214, 215
    ambient, 71, 136
    asbestos in, 43, 74, 76, 100, 169, 177
    breathing, 39, 77, 80
    concentration of, 76
    controlling, 73, 74, 81, 98, 136
    industrial, 158, 159
    nuisance, 70, 73–74, 87, 104, 206
    problems with, 63, 80, 81, 106
    sampling, 172, 209
    vermiculite and, 70
    Zonolite, 156
Dust control equipment, 73, 81

Eaton, Fred, 166
Economic problems, 72, 89, 214–15
Egan, Thomas: on Selikoff, 163
Egilman, David, 54, 57
    Grace and, 52–53, 61
    papers of, 53, 55–56
Egilman, Felix, 57
Ellman, Philip: on pulmonary asbestosis, 99
Emphysema, 77, 114
Engineering News-Record, 165
Engle, Rudolph, 77
Environmentalists, 24, 129, 130, 195, 217
Environmental laws, 148, 194
Environmental Protection Agency (EPA), 85, 92, 132–33, 154, 169
    asbestos and, 24, 69, 145, 146, 163, 170, 174
    authority of, 135, 171
    criticism of, 204
    Gayla and, 200, 201
    Grace and, 93, 199, 206–10, 213, 215
    letters to, 195
    Libby and, 72, 151–52, 220–21
    Monokote-3 and, 167
    occupational safety and, 149
    OIG and, 144–45
    OSHA and, 172
    Peronard and, 150
    Power and, 21
    Racicot and, 123
    sampling by, 69, 71, 144, 169, 176
    schools and, 163–64
    Scotts Company and, 137–38

Superfund and, 199
TSCA and, 144
vermiculite and, 121, 221
WTC disaster and, 155–56, 171, 176, 177, 179
Zonolite and, 22
Epidemiological studies, 140
Eschenbach, Harry, 66, 73, 103, 107, 110, 167
    deposition by, 90
    Irons and, 108, 109
    on Scotts situation, 140
Euclid dump trucks, 36, 40
Euston, Greg, 212
Exposure, 80, 98, 114, 123, 136, 143, 175, 206, 214
    asbestosis and, 135
    health effects of, 159–60
    limiting, 83
    nonoccupational, 173, 174
    occupational, 122, 138
    rates of, 120
    tremolite, 207

Fairness in Asbestos Compensation Act, 122
Favorito, Mario, 141
FBI, Grace and, 54–55
Fiber counts, 83–84, 135, 159, 176
Fiberglass, 157
Fibrosis, 67, 97, 113, 120
    asbestos and, 100, 119
    kinds of, 119
    tremolite and, 109
Fields, Willis: lung disease for, 77
Fireproofing, 156, 169
    asbestos, 60, 166
    binding, 164
    non-asbestos, 166, 168
    vermiculite and, 165
Fiscus, Lloyd, 78
Fishing, 72, 221
Flathead Lake, 23, 100
Flathead Monitor, on Alley, 32–33
Flathead River, 23
Flathead Valley, 23–24, 100
Ford Motor Company, 34
Fortune 500, Grace and, 51
Fortune magazine, on lawsuits, 210
Franks, asbestos and, 96
Fresenius Medical Care Holdings, 211
Funerals, 107

Gardner, Le Roy, 160, 161, 162
Gas chambers, 58
Gay, Murray, 33
Geiger, Heather, 84
Geiger, Randy, 83, 85
    asbestos levels and, 83–84
General Services Administration, WTC and, 176

Genetic research, 119
Gidley, Jim: death of, 182
Gidley, Louise, 182, 183
Glacier National Park, 23, 68, 150
Grace, J. Peter, 51, 52
    Ambrose and, 59, 60–61
    animosity for, 50
    bureaucracy and, 142
    chemical business and, 57
    Dewey and Almy and, 63
    Nazis and, 56–57
    Reagan and, 60, 142, 144
Grace, James: lineage of, 51
Grace, John, 51
Grace, Joseph Peter, 51
Grace, Michael, 50, 51
Grace, Morgan, 51
Grace, William Russell, 50, 51
    scandal for, 52
Grace Chemicals, 57
Grace Commission, 52, 54, 60, 142, 145
Grace Line ships, 53, 54
Granger, Hugh, 172, 176, 177, 178
Great Northern Railroad, 33
Ground Zero
    asbestos at, 170, 171, 178
    dust at, 169
    testing/sampling at, 172
Guzman Tellez, Julio, 55–56
Gypsum, 164

Hardy, Bruce, 95, 105
Health agencies, asbestos-related diseases and, 118
Health issues, 12, 134, 137, 151, 156, 183
Health insurance, 7, 49, 173
Health Science Center (University of Texas), 116
Heart problems, 97, 181
Hendrickson, Ed: lung disease for, 78
HEPA-filtered air purifiers, 157
HEPA vacuum, 156
Hi-Line, 23, 147
Hill, Rick, 122
Hill, Robert, 132
Hillis, Bill, 33–34
Hitler, Adolf, 57, 58
Holian, Andrij, 118, 119, 120
    lung biology and, 121
    research by, 115, 116, 117
Holiday, Bob: on Zonolite, 34
Hoover, J. Edgar, 54, 55
Hospice program, 106, 107, 205
Hot Springs, 100
House fill, 34
Howard, Joseph Kinsey, 31
Howell, Verle, 203–4
HP Environmental, 172
Hunt, Linda, 57, 59, 62
Hunting, 72, 129
Hygiene, 83, 173

I.G. Farben, 57, 59
Immune system, 119
    asbestos and, 120–21
Industrial Accident Board, 82
Industrial Disease Act, 81
Industrial Hygiene Act (1939),
    131
Industrial Hygiene
    Foundation, 159
Industrial Revolution, 96
Inhalers, 14, 115
Inspections, 36, 75–76,
    136–37, 150, 167
Institute for Occupational
    Medicine, 196
Institute of Industrial
    Medicine, 161
Insulation, 60, 143, 152
    binding, 164
    removal of, 145, 212
    spray-on, 164
    vermiculite, 71, 118
    Zonolite, 21, 121, 122, 207,
    212, 221, 221n
Insurance companies, 81, 82, 83
Interior Department, Racicot
    and, 147
Intrapleural tests, 108
Irons, Karen, 105, 111
Irons, Kirsten, 112
Irons, Richard, 95, 103, 104–5,
    107, 111, 185
    addiction treatment center
    and, 112
    deposition by, 186
    Eschenbach and, 108, 109
    pilot project and, 205
    practice problems for, 110
    self-interest of, 105

Jacobs, Mr., 133
JAMA. See Journal of the
    American Medical
    Association
Jannot, Mark, 178, 179
Jaycees, Lovick and, 35
Jenkins, Cate, 170, 171, 177
J. Neils Lumber Company, 124
Johns-Manville Corporation,
    108, 109, 158, 159, 160,
    162, 210
Journal of Industrial Hygiene, 99
Journal of Pathology, 98
Journal of the American Medical
    Association (JAMA), 88,
    97
    on lung cancer/asbestos, 99
Judge, Don, 134, 150

Kair, Morissa: lung disease for,
    78
Kalispell, 23, 27, 28, 43, 68
Kalispell Daily Inter Lake, 193
KDC. See Kootenai
    Development Company
Kelley, Joseph, 80–81
Kempski, Hans, 55

King Copper, 130, 131
Knights of Malta, 52
Kootenai Clinic, 105
Kootenai Development
    Company (KDC), 209
Kootenai Indians, 1
Kootenai National Forest, 68
Kootenai River, 1, 3, 10, 23,
    31, 90, 180, 218
    mine waste in, 69
    storage facility on, 36
Kootenai Valley Products Co.,
    33
Kostic, Peter, 76, 80
Kujawa, Ray: lung disease for,
    77

La Casa de Amigos, 201, 202
Lady Inspectors, 96–97
Lake Koocanusa, 23
Lantos, Tom: on
    Grace/Ambrose, 60–61
Lanza, Anthony, 161–62
Larrick, S. Y.: letter by, 82
Latency period, 97
Lavage, 119
Lawn and garden chemicals,
    137–38, 143
Lawsuits, 12–13, 113, 182,
    183, 184, 205, 209–10
    asbestos, 51, 52, 212
    class action, 212
    tobacco, 53, 56
    wrongful-death, 18, 185,
    187, 189
Lee Enterprises, 126–27, 148
Leukemia, 113
Levine, Louis, 126
Liability, 83
Libby
    air sampling in, 144
    as America's Chernobyl, 150
    anomaly of, 29
    betrayal of, 194
    described, 23, 118
    economy of, 72, 89
    EPA and, 151–52
    Grace and, 62–63, 64, 199
    isolation of, 24–25
    labor in, 131
    maps of, 72
Libby Creek, 3, 10
Libby dam, 25, 65, 179, 180
Libby Hospital, 108
Libby Hotel, 33
Libby Loggers, 23, 131
Lincoln County, 24
    asbestos in, 215
    cleanup in, 212
    population of, 25
    revenue bonds by, 81
Lions Club, Lovick and, 35
Little, William, 102
    on asbestos/Libby, 100
    Lovick and, 100, 101
    X rays and, 101, 110
Locke, Robert, 140–41, 142

Lockey, Jim, 138–39
Lockheed, 62
Logging, 27, 29, 68, 105, 129,
    222
    decline in, 150
    restrictions on, 72
London Underground, Grace
    and, 169
Lovick, Bonnie, 35, 153
Lovick, Earl, 46, 74, 79, 103,
    128, 140, 153
    on asbestos, 38
    on Craver, 80
    death of, 35, 65, 77
    on discharge, 71
    funerals and, 107
    on Grace, 76
    inspectors and, 133
    Irons and, 106
    Little and, 100, 101
    lung disease for, 77, 78
    Margaret on, 17
    moral obligation and, 182
    on plaquing, 89
    popularity of, 35
    testimony of, 36, 37, 77
    Thomson and, 9
    Wilkins and, 86–87
    Zonolite and, 35–36
Lung cancer, 13, 67, 107, 141,
    182
    asbestos-inspired, 9, 77, 99
    chrysotile and, 162
    deaths from, 88, 99
    developing, 99, 114
    misdiagnosis of, 12
    treating, 113
Lung disease, 106, 107, 207
    asbestos-related, 37, 77–78,
    113, 117, 152
    environmental, 117
    evidence of, 102
Lung function tests, 64, 78,
    102–3
Lutheran Church, Irons and,
    106

MacKenzie, Robert, 6, 84
Maclean, Norman, 130
Madison River, 180
Malone, Michael
    on Butte, 125
    on copper mining, 125–26
    on Montana Power
    Company, 126
    on Racicot, 147
Manganese, 120
Manifest Destiny, 30
Man-lifts, 79, 80
Maps, rural Montana, 71–72
Martin-Marietta, 62
Martz, Judy
    Gayla on, 155, 217
    Libby and, 198, 199,
    213–14, 216
    Peronard and, 213, 214
    Superfund and, 216

Maryland Casualty Company, 82, 83
Masonry Fill, 167, 169
Maximum allowable concentration, 75, 131
Mayo, William B., 34
McCaig, Bill, 73, 84, 103, 128
  Darko and, 129
  funerals and, 107
  Grace and, 183
  Irons and, 106
  moral obligation and, 182
McCullough, Warren, 195
McGarvey, Allan, 211
McGarvey, Dale, 183, 184, 188
McGarvey, Heberling and Sullivan (law firm), 184
McGill University, research at, 141
McGrath, Mike, 127, 217
McNair, Louise, 65–66
McNair, Michael: death of, 65–66
McQueen, Rose, 26
Media, 201, 202–3
Medical Board, 158
Medical care, 12, 14, 17–18, 221
  applying for, 207
Medical insurance, 103
Medical plan, 207, 216
Medicare, 115
MEIC. *See* Montana Environmental Information Center
Mellon Institute of Industrial Research, 158
Memorial Gymnasium, Racicot at, 124
Mental health, 187
Mesabi Iron Range, 47
Mesothelial cells, 113, 114
Mesothelioma, 9, 67, 107, 109, 114
  latency period for, 149
Methyl cellulose filters, 171
Metropolitan Life, 159
Microns, 172
Militia of Montana, 24
Miller, Holly, 195, 196
Milling equipment, 37
Milltown Dam, 127
Miners' Union Hall, 126
Mine Safety and Health Administration (MSHA), 86, 136–37
Mine sites, reclamation of, 127
Mint Bar, 184
Miron, Fred, 47–49
  asbestosis for, 49
Miron, Paul, 47–49
  asbestosis for, 49
  Vietnam and, 47, 49
Molloy, Donald: Grace/EPA and, 209–10
Monokote, 60, 168, 174
  formula for, 165–66

Monokote-3, 165
  banning, 167
  chrysotile and, 166
  recipe for, 164
Monokote-4, 166, 167, 168
Montague, Murray, 97
Montana: A Contemporary Profile (Malone), 147
Montana Constitution (1972), 127
Montana Environmental Information Center (MEIC), 192
Montana: High, Wide and Handsome (Howard), 31
Montana Human Rights Network, 24
Montana Mining Association, 129, 131
Montana Power Company, 126
Montana Supreme Court, 183
Moonsuits, 214, 215
Moral obligation, 52, 83, 182
Morris, Roger, 190, 191, 208
Morrison, Allen, 164
Mortality, analysis of, 107
Mother Jones, story in, 73
Mt. Everest, Irons and, 111
Mt. Sinai Hospital, 88, 162
MSHA. *See* Mine Safety and Health Administration
Multibestos, 63
Mushroom season, 72, 91, 92, 221

Nadler, Jerry, 176
National Emission Standard for Asbestos law, 164
National Geographic Adventure, 178
National Institute for Occupation Safety and Health (NIOSH)
  asbestos and, 163
  Grace and, 139–40, 141, 142
  haggling with, 143
  occupational safety and, 149
  Scotts and, 139–40
National Institute of Health, 118
National Medical Care, 211
Nazi Corridor, 24
Nazis/Nazi sympathizers, 61
  Grace and, 52–54, 56, 57
Neils, Julius, 29, 32, 89
Nelson, Floyd E.: espionage by, 54–55
Nelson, Les: on evil, 38
Nelson, Woodrow: respiratory function tests and, 102
Nerve gas, 58
Never Again Consulting, 52
Newark Evening News, 165
New York Department of Health, 176

New York Times, 168, 181, 211
  Libby and, 201
  on WTC/asbestos, 155
New York University, Institute of Industrial Medicine at, 161
NIOSH. *See* National Institute for Occupation Safety and Health
Nitrate of soda, 51
Noranda, bid by, 130
Norris, Paul, 73, 153, 206
  on allegations, 70
  income of, 181
  on lawsuits, 210
Nuremberg trials, 59

Occupational Disease Act (1959), 82, 101, 131, 183
Occupational safety, 122, 149
Occupational Safety and Health Administration (OSHA), 146, 173, 174, 175
  asbestos and, 135, 163
  EPA and, 172
  occupational safety and, 149
  regulations by, 89, 135
  testing by, 138
Office of Inspector General (OIG), 136, 137, 146
  EPA and, 144–45
Oklahoma City bombing, 49
Oliverio, Bob, 78, 109
O.M. Scott and Sons, health crisis for, 137–38
O.M. Scott Company, 89, 144
Osteomyelitis, 111
Owen-Corning Fiberglass, 159
Oxygen deprivation, asbestosis and, 16

Panagra, 54, 55
Parenchyma, 120
Parker, Lerah, 90–91
  asbestos and, 92
  exposure for, 93
  nursery of, 209, 215
  stipend for, 93
Parker, Mel, 90, 91, 94
  asbestos and, 92
  nursery of, 209, 215
  stipend for, 93
Particulates, 135, 157
Patagonia outlet store, 194, 195
Pend Oreille lake system, 24
People Magazine, 201
Permissible Exposure Limits (PEL), 137
Peronard, Paul, 74, 93, 137, 144, 146, 173, 198, 204, 207–8
  on asbestos, 150
  characteristics of, 72
  cynicism of, 145
  EPA and, 150, 213
  Gayla and, 200, 201

on Grace, 209
listing and, 199
Martz and, 213, 214, 217
media and, 201
Parkers and, 215
public trust for, 151
report by, 149
tasks of, 72–73
technical aspects and, 201
Phase contrast microscopy,
    174, 175, 176, 201
problems with, 84
Pioneer Society, 25
Pleural effusions, 114, 138, 139
Pleural plaquing, 9, 13, 88, 89,
    113
Pneumoconiosis, 77, 158, 161
Pneumoconiosis Bureau, 161
Pneumonia, 15
Polycarbonate fibers, 171
Port Authority of New York, 164
Potassium, 14
Power, Georgina, 20
Power, Mike, 20–21, 22
Processing, 34, 36, 39, 79, 132,
    143
dry, 80, 98
Project National Interest, 59, 62
Project Paperclip, 57
Protective equipment, 169–70,
    173, 175, 178
Public Citizen, 103
Public Health Department,
    report by, 75
Publicity, 202–3, 209
Pulmonary function tests, 106,
    150
Pulmonary infections, 150

Quebec Asbestos Mining
    Association, 161
"Quebec Asbestos Workers"
    (file), 161

Racicot, Marc, 122, 198
asbestos problems and, 121
criticism of, 147, 148, 151
EPA and, 123
Libby and, 124, 125, 131
political skills of, 147–48
roots of, 124
water quality laws and, 129
Railroads, 29, 33, 69, 72
Raintree Nursery, 90, 208, 215
Rainy Creek, 68, 90, 106, 192
memorial at, 222
vermiculite from, 30
Rainy Creek Road, 65, 69–70,
    179, 203, 207, 214, 215
Raish, Bob, 133
Rales, 114
Raybestos Manhattan, 159
Reagan, Ronald, 60, 62, 148,
    180
Grace and, 51, 52, 54, 142,
    144, 145
Real estate market, 129, 203–4

Recipes, Zonolite, 32
Reclamation projects, 206
Reforestation projects, 91
Regulations, 145, 166
mining, 135
unions and, 99
water quality, 130
Rehberg, Denny, 201
Reishi project, 94
Reppe, Walter, 57
Republican National
    Committee, Racicot and,
    124, 198
Rescue workers, protective
    equipment for, 169–70
Respirators, 39, 73, 80, 136,
    156, 170, 175, 178, 179
Respiratory function tests, 77,
    102
Respiratory problems, 102,
    141, 175
Revenue Oversight
    Committee, 128
Rexall Drug Store, 202
Rhode Island Monthly, 57
Rice, Greg, 105
River Wild, The (film), 23
Robinson, Dave, 41, 42
Rocky Mountains, 23, 72, 129,
    209
Roofing, 32
Roosevelt, Teddy, 51
Rosenberg, Arnold, 56–57
Rotary Club, Irons and, 106
R.T. Vanderbilt Company, 108,
    109
Ryan, John D.: Montana
    Power Company and, 126
Ryan, Royce, 179, 180, 212

Safety committee, Lovick and,
    37–38
Safety violations, 136–37
St. Johns Lutheran Hospital,
    96, 207
Santa Lucia (ship), 54
Saranac Institute, 160
Saranac Laboratory, 159–60, 161
Sarin, 58
Scanning electron microscopy,
    174
Schepers, Gerrit, 160, 161, 162
Schlichtman, Jan, 184
Schneider, Andrew, 192, 194,
    221n
death certificates and, 206
Gayla and, 191, 193
Miller and, 195
Schools, asbestos in, 71,
    163–64, 171, 214
Scotts Company, 90, 143
EPA and, 137–38
health crisis for, 137–38
NIOSH and, 139–40
Screenings, 81, 207
Sealed Air, 211
Seattle Post-Intelligencer, 192

Sebastien, Patrick, 66
Secret Agenda (Hunt), 57
Sedler, Laura: pilot project
    and, 205
Selikoff, Irving, 99, 108
Egan on, 163
study by, 88, 89, 163
warnings by, 179
Settlements, 12–13, 82, 182,
    185, 187, 188
asbestos-related, 146
winning, 183
Shareholder distributions, 81,
    85, 210–11, 212
Siegner, Cathy, 129, 130
Sierra Club, Irons and, 110
Silica, 74, 96
Silicates, 96
Silicon, 96
Silicon dioxide, 96
Silicosis, 81, 96, 103
asbestosis and, 97
Simonich, Mark, 122, 123, 129
Skramstad, Brady, 43, 44, 45
Skramstad, Brent, 43, 44
asbestosis for, 45, 184
Skramstad, Gayla, 41, 44, 47,
    191
Skramstad, Laurel, 27, 44
asbestosis for, 45, 184
Skramstad, Les, 27, 42, 62,
    185, 186, 189
anger of, 45, 68
asbestos project and, 41, 86
award for, 184
children of, 43, 46, 47
deposition for, 36, 46
diabetes for, 44
diagnosis for, 114
Dillon and, 196
as dump boss, 40–41
Gayla and, 46, 154, 183, 184
introduction to, 67
lawsuit by, 102–3, 187
Martz and, 217
Morris and, 191
on Racicot, 148
settlement for, 25–26
Whitehouse and, 113
at Zonolite, 39–40, 43
Skramstad, Norita Gardiner,
    41, 47, 62, 67, 68, 184,
    185, 189, 208
anger of, 45
children of, 43, 44–45
Dillon and, 196
Gayla and, 28, 154
lawsuit by, 187
on Les, 26, 46
Libby and, 27, 43
Skramstad, Sloan, 44, 45
Smith, Dale, 40
Smith, William, 108–9
Smoking
asbestos and, 88, 89, 99, 163
ban on, 88–89
stopping, 89, 106

Snowshoe Peak, 110
Social Security, Ryan and, 180, 181
Society for Occupational and Environmental Health, 108
Soil testing, 149
Sophie, 53, 61, 62
Spence, Michael, 148, 149
Spin-offs, 211, 212
Spokane Airport, expansion of, 167
Standards, 135
    air quality, 132, 133–34
    asbestos, 138
    health, 158–59
    industry, 75
Stansbury Holding Corporation, 194, 196
Steel, asbestos and, 169
Streep, Meryl, 23
Stringer, Alan, 78, 80, 90, 202
    on allegations, 70
    controversy and, 73
    on medical coverage, 207
    on rights, 208
Strip-mining, 36
"Study of the Interior Fire Protection Requirements of the Exterior Columns for the World Trade Center Project" (Grace), 165
Sullivan, Roger, 154–55, 184, 186, 211, 212
    on lawsuits, 183
Superfund, 127, 200, 201, 204, 218
    EPA and, 199
    Martz and, 198–99, 216
    National Priorities List, 217
    Zonolite and, 221
Support group, 205
Swenson, Gary, v, 11
Swenson, Jenan, 122, 155, 189, 203, 216
    adulthood of, 10–11
    on caregiving, 16
    DeShazers and, 218–19
    Gayla and, 154
    journey of, 219–20
    Margaret and, 18–19, 219
Synthetic rubber, 58

Tabun, 58
Tailings, 69, 81, 85, 214–15
Tax Appeals Board, 128
Taxation of the Mines in Montana, The (Levine), 126
TEM. *See* Transmission electron microscopy
Terra-lite, 35
Terrorist attacks, 155–56, 170
Textile mills, 98
Theo-Dur capsules, 14
Thompson Falls, 24, 203

Thomson, Dale, 6, 7
    asbestosis and, 9
    death of, 9–10, 15
    management and, 8, 9
Thomson, Eva, 8, 28, 81
    on COPD, 9
    on Dale's death, 9–10
    Gayla and, 4, 6, 154
    lawsuit by, 185, 187
    medical expenses and, 17–18
    mother and, 3, 15
    on school, 3
    settlement and, 187, 188, 189
Thorn, Orville, 41
Threshold limit value (TLV), 135, 136
Tobacco companies, suing, 53, 56
Toole, Ken, 24
Torkelson, Gordon: death of, 40–41
Town meeting, 216
Toxic Substances Control Act (TSCA), 144
Toxic tort cases, 56
Trans-tracheal scoop, 14
Transmission electron microscopy (TEM), 174, 175, 176, 201
Tremolite, 36–38, 63, 64, 66, 69, 86, 101, 120, 132, 134, 143
    asbestos and, 100, 195
    cancer/fibrosis and, 109
    crystalline-structured, 196
    defining, 87
    exposure to, 207
    information about, 106
    studying, 107, 108–9
    vermiculite and, 109
Trudeau Institute, 159
TSCA. *See* Toxic Substances Control Act
Tuberculosis, 77, 98
20/20, 201

"Uncivil Action, An" (Schneider), 193
Underwriters' Laboratories, 166
Unions, asbestos regulations and, 99
U.S. Army Counterintelligence Corps, 110
U.S. Bureau of Mines, 135, 143, 146, 163
U.S. Bureau of Reclamation, 26
U.S. Department of Energy, 62
U.S. Forest Service
    Irons and, 110
    McNair and, 65
    reforestation projects by, 91
    Skramstad and, 26
U.S. Geological Survey, on vermiculite, 30

U.S. Public Health Service, 75–76, 159
U.S. State Department, 54
Universal Zonolite Insulation Company
    Alley and, 20, 33
    benefits at, 42–43
    death at, 40–41
    emissions at, 167
    Grace and, 35, 37, 51, 60, 62, 76, 77, 102, 167
    Hillis and, 33–34
    McNair and, 65
    ore at, 34
    problem at, 73–74, 80, 81, 89
    Skramstad at, 28, 29
    Vatland at, 6
University of Maryland, Nazi documents at, 54
University of Montana, 153
    research at, 116, 119

Vatland, Margaret
    anger of, 17, 19
    death of, 15–16, 19, 219
    deposition of, 12
    Gayla and, 7, 10, 12, 14–19
    health problems for, 10, 12–15, 18–19
    Jenan and, 11
    Perley and, 2
    settlement for, 12–13
    workmen's compensation for, 6
Vatland, Perley, 1, 7, 19, 27
    Dale and, 8
    death of, 2, 6, 8, 10, 81
    Gayla on, 5
    Margaret on, 17
    music and, 28
    possessions of, 3
Veltman, Preston, 60
Vermiculite, 33, 39, 75, 92, 115, 148
    asbestos and, 42, 90, 139, 194
    as base material, 34–35
    deposits of, 30
    EPA and, 121, 221
    export of, 35
    fireproofing with, 165
    grade 3, 164, 166
    high-grade, 64
    mining, 62, 70, 143, 146, 194–97
    playground, 189
    as potting soil, 35
    processing, 36, 39, 79, 132, 143
    tremolite and, 109
    working with, 118
Vermiculite and Asbestos Co., 33
Vermiculite-gypsum plaster, 165
Vermiculite Mountain, 38, 67, 68, 156

Veterans Administration, 49
Victims, 122, 181, 203, 215
  bankruptcy and, 210
  memorial for, 222
  support group for, 205
Vining, Rod, 166
Vorwald, Arthur, 160–61, 162

Wahl, Betsy, 146
Wake, Ben, 77, 82, 98
  departure of, 131–32
  industry standards and, 75
  report by, 74–75, 76, 80
Walpole plant, 64
Walter, Dave, 24
Wardell, John: asbestos
  problem and, 146
Water quality, 127, 129, 130,
  169
Weis, Chris, 149, 156, 165,
  170, 199
  calculations of, 166
  on exposure, 214
  technical aspects and, 201
  on tremolite asbestos, 69
  Vermiculite Mountain and,
  68
Welch, Lilas "Shorty," 81,
  82–83
Western News, 89, 90, 190
  on Alley, 33
  Stringer in, 208
  on Terra-lite, 35
Wet mill, 49, 81, 83
Whitehouse, Alan, 87–88, 92,
  112, 181
  on asbestos exposure, 114
  on asbestosis, 115

  on fibrosis, 113
  testimony by, 102–3
White Lung program, 115
Whitman, Christine Todd,
  155, 170, 176
  on air/water quality, 169
Whole Wheat Zonobread,
  recipe for, 32
Wilderness Act, 131
Wilkins, Bob, 38
  on Banks, 142
  on Craver, 79
  Lovick and, 86–87
  lung capacity and, 88
  on showers, 85
  on test results, 79
Winter, asbestosis and, 46–47
Wolter, Jack, 109, 209
Woman's Club, 29
Wood, Chip, 168
Wood, E. S., 89
Workers' compensation law, 6,
  82, 158, 182
World Trade Center (WTC)
  asbestos at, 155, 156–57,
  164–65, 166, 169, 176,
  177–78
  EPA and, 155–56, 171–72
  Grace and, 152, 164–65
W.R. Grace & Company, 2, 4,
  8, 38, 74, 91
  antagonists for, 52–53
  departure of, 190, 191, 192
  EPA and, 93, 199, 206,
  207–8, 209–10, 213, 215
  fighting, 46
  formation of, 50
  legacy of, 151–52, 192

  revenues for, 64
  South America and, 55–56
  strategy by, 140–41
  subsidiaries of, 51
  "W.R. Grace Bankruptcy
  Newsletter," 210

X rays, 37, 64, 99, 103, 106,
  110, 114, 115
  asbestos fibers and, 101
  chest, 77, 78, 79
  reading, 100, 101–2, 108

Yaak River, 205
Yang, Julie, 73, 84
Yellowstone National Park,
  130, 147
Yellowtail, Bill, 146

Zonolite, 72, 74, 98, 102, 134,
  148, 166
  asbestos and, 20, 63, 168
  exporting, 32
  King Copper and, 131
  mining, 36
  recipes with, 32
  report on, 74–75
  shipping, 33
  touting of, 31–32
Zonolite Canyon, 65
Zonolite Company. *See*
  Universal Zonolite
  Insulation Company
Zonolite insulation, 21, 121,
  122, 207, 212, 221, 221n
Zonolite Mountain, 71
Zyklon-B, 58